D1429007

Depression and Globalization

Carl Walker

Depression and Globalization
The Politics of Mental Health in the 21ˢᵗ Century

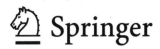
Springer

Carl Walker
School of Applied Social Science
University of Brighton
Mayfield House
Falmer
Brighton BN1 9PH
c.j.walker@brighton.ac.uk

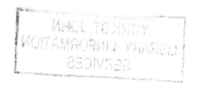

ISBN: 978-0-387-72712-7   e-ISBN: 978-0-387-72723-4

Library of Congress Control Number: 2007934982

Printed on acid-free paper.

9 8 7 6 5 4 3 2 1

springer.com

For pap, a better man I have yet to meet

Preface

Why Depression and Why Now?

When I sat down to write a book on how recent global political changes are contributing to our current prevalence and understanding of depression, a colleague and good friend asked 'why now?' The implication was that depression had been around for a great many years and had been a problem for people whose task it was to address it for every bit as long. The reason why I wanted to write about depression now was straightforward. Stated simply, an increasing number of people are suffering from depression as the years pass and in a medical context it is almost universally agreed that its status as a health issue is now paramount. Depression is now considered to be one of the most serious health issues faced in Europe[1] and the United States in particular. In the UK and US, the cost of adult depression is believed to be in the region of 15.5 billion euros and 100 billion euros, respectively. In recent years, there has been a growing understanding of the immense burden that the illness imposes on both individuals, their friends and families, and their communities and it now represents 4.4% of the total disease burden around the world, in the same range as heart disease.[2] Whereas in 1990, depressive disorders were estimated to be the leading cause of disability and were the fourth leading cause of total global burden of disease; the World Health Organisation expect them to be the second leading cause of disease burden by 2020.

So why is the disease burden of depression predicted to increase? I hope that, through the course of this book, the reader will come to better understand the everyday relevance of the political, economic and social changes that we have nebulously come to understand as globalization and the increased incidence of depression in the western world. In 1979, something happened in the US and the UK that did not happen all over the world. An interconnected set of social, economic and political changes occurred that placed a grinding halt on the post-war social democratic consensus. For this reason, this book focuses mainly on the changes that occurred in the US and the UK and the effects that they wrought. With the possible exception of New Zealand, nowhere else in the developed world experienced such an almighty shift to the right as when the neoliberal project took hold in the US and the UK.

In many ways the 1980s and 1990s exhibited a veritable simulation of early nineteenth century free-market economics. The rebirth of the new right in the 1970s championed economic liberalism and while the changes were felt most profoundly in the UK and the US, these countries were far from unique in their exposure to this newly rampant liberalism. In country upon country, markets were deregulated, state planning and power dismantled, welfare was cut and/or criminalized and full employment policies abandoned.

We have witnessed an era of free-market fundamentalism where such economic conjectures as supply side and trickle down economics have been celebrated as panaceas for a declining social order. A war on regulation has led to a disproportionate increase in the needs of the business community and such perspectives have been supported by the clandestine decision making of international financial bodies like the World Bank and the IMF. These political and fiscal developments have contributed to a growth in social inequality and (of the developed countries) this inequality has been most pronounced in the US and the UK. Between the late 1970s and late 1990s, the average income for US families in the bottom fifth of the income scale fell by 5%, whereas that of the top families rose by 33%. The numbers of people in poverty in the UK increased from 5 m to 14.1 m between 1979 and 1992 and in the US a conservative (very conservative according to some sources) estimate of over 31 m Americans currently live below the poverty line (11.3% of the population) with 41% of those having less than half the official income of the poverty line.

I will create a context for defining the structures and practices associated with globalization, their genesis and the ways in which they have developed in recent years. Such economic and political structures are not simply nebulous dynamics that lurk around the backwaters of our growing prevalence of mental health issues, they are the key factors. The political and social changes of the New Right profoundly influenced a number of mental health issues but this book specifically concerns the depressive disorders. It concerns the way that these political and economic changes relate not only to the number of people who are living with depression but the way that we have come to understand and treat it.

The Psychological Sciences, Depressions and Definitions

I will also contextualize the mental health industry and the psychological sciences by placing them in the recent political, social and economic events discussed above. The status of the psychological sciences, as they stand, is generally incoherent and introspective. We have focused too much on the individualistic and dispositional factors that we feel we can control and neglected the social and political context within which we all operate. Psychiatrists, for example, come to their work following prolonged tuition in physical medicine and naturally tend towards a physical basis for disorders.

I discuss how a mistrust of the non-scientific, a protection of funding imperatives and an almost absolute refusal to reflect on their status as a discursive approach has led the psychological sciences towards a paradoxical territory where their systems of treatment and therapies also represent tacit support for the political system that creates such harmful circumstances in the first place. Despite a wide body of research implicating the role of social and economic factors, social scientists still tend to focus on the psychology of the individual as the unit of investigation and this approach has been rewarded in the current economic and political climate. Material interests underpin cultural power and the 'depression industry' is as responsive to these interests as other industries.

Throughout the book I will talk about depression but by using the term 'depression' I would like to make the point that I am not necessarily subscribing to the school of thought that considers depression a unitary disease concept. Rather I refer to the psychosocial and biological distress and difficulties that we have come to understand as depressive disorders. When I talk about the research I will tend to use the language used by the researchers themselves. By discussing 'clinical depression' or 'major depression' I do not, by definition, rule out multiple concepts. It is far from accepted truth that there is one depressive disease and this will be discussed further in the first two chapters where I relate our understanding of classifications of mental illness and depression to political pressures in recent history. While the clinical relevance of the classification procedure may be debated, the diagnostic symptom guide can be useful as a proxy for the suffering and distress that we have come to understand as depression.

The more one becomes familiar with the research literature on depression the more complex the illness can seem. One thing we can be sure of is that depression is not a minor ailment that can be 'shrugged off'. It can be a life-wrecking, hideously painful illness for sufferers and their families. This understanding of depression is not shared by many as there is often a tendency to understand the illness as little more than feeling 'down in the dumps'. Such attitudes to depression are discussed with respect to our understandings of mental distress through history and how the stigma associated with depression has come to be generated and maintained in our era.

A Few Final Comments…

This is a book on the illness of depression first and foremost and as such I have used Chapter 1 to try to cover what we have come to understand by this term. Readers may come to this book from a number of different walks of life and through academic or non-academic backgrounds. They will have different experiences of what it means to be depressed either through their own experience, the experience of those close to them or other sources. They may have experience of depression from an academic or voluntary sector context or may not be familiar with depression and so it is important for me to use the first chapter to try to give an overview of what different people mean by depression. I have tried to give a sense of what it can be like to live with the illness both as a sufferer and as a family or friend, as an adult and as a child, and how the mental health sciences and medical establishment have come to define the illness and the ramifications of these descriptions. Some elements of this description and explanation will be familiar to some readers but is necessary in order that we provide a detailed grounding for subsequent chapters that provide a more historical and integrated context for depression.

With regards to the main body of the book, I hope that the views, research, facts and conjecture contained within take the form of constructive criticism. Mental health is an area within which many people have worked to try to alleviate the suffering of so many others. As such, I hope that the views within are seen less as an attack than as an appreciation of some of the limitations of past work that has served to constrain our understanding of mental illness in certain ways. I apologize in advance for those who may take some of the points in this book as personal attacks on their work and their character. This was never my intention. There is a grey area that exists in the social sciences where practitioners, with the greatest intentions in the world, reinforce hegemonic ideologies that serve to both benefit and denigrate their clients concurrently. This paradox lies at the heart of much of the work in the psychological sciences and while I cannot claim to have the torch-light that will lead us through this tunnel, I can try to urge social scientists to be more reflective about their work in historical, political and economic contexts.

It is my belief that this subject needs both a microscopic and macroscopic perspective and that it requires the crossing of a number of academic boundaries. It needs to draw on social sciences, medicine, the media, economics, politics and history in order to understand the interconnecting relationships between the different factors that influence our approaches to mental health and depression. It is my firm belief that, if we are to truly understand the economic and structural decisions that affect public health imperatives in the twenty-first century, a more broad ranging focus will need to be adopted.

This book is not a science book in the traditional manner. I have used the evidence to build the case relating political and economic changes to depression prevalence but there is no smoking gun. If you are seeking definitive answers then this is the wrong book. There is conjecture and suggestions and possibilities and I believe that these combine to create a convincing case and one that is rarely considered in the modern mental health sciences. Those whose lives have been affected by depression and whose lives will be affected in the future deserve to be given the whole story. This has not always been forthcoming in previous literature.

Finally, this book will not tell you how to recover from depression. It will tell you how the political and economic organization of Western societies and, particularly the US and the UK, play a role in increasing the likelihood that people will become depressed. We need a debate about depression and we need one fast, because it is becoming the number one public health concern of the World Health Organization. We need a debate about what it is, how it is treated, and how we understand depression in relation to the changing shape of society. We have to understand better the consequences of how we, as public and health professionals alike, contribute to the shame, guilt and stigma experienced by so many people. Political, social and economic structures are not discourses that exist in a vacuum, hermetically sealed from the psychological or medical 'worlds' of depression. They are forces that fundamentally constrain the suffering and distress that people have to endure. This book places depression in the context of its political and economic history, to redress a balance that has contributed to its shifting precipitously close to a psychiatric epidemic.

Carl Walker

Acknowledgments

This work has been written over the last three years and to do so while holding down a full-time job requires the understanding and sacrifice of a number of people.

Firstly, and most importantly, I would like to thank my wife Ruth for being an unending source of inspiration, encouragement and tolerance over this period of time. Not just the practical help but the constant support and sacrifice without which I would not have been able to write this book or develop a career in mental health. This book is a result of her generosity.

I would like to reserve special thanks to Jan Wilde, Justin Walker, Adrian Walker and Christine McConville, my family, for their love and support.

I would also like to thank Gareth Griffiths, a good friend whose intellectual acuity and generous spirit allowed me to open up to a new understanding of psychology and mental health. I would like to thank Jerry Byrne for his knowing how important it is that we open up a debate.

I would like to thank Linda Papadopoulos for giving me the chance to work in mental health and Michael King and Irwin Nazareth for helping me to become a better academic.

Thanks also to Paul Hitchcock, Lee Myring, Mickey Dolenz, Jon Hayes, Iain Salvage, Nicola Hitchcock, Marie Myring, Siva Ganeshanandan, Kelvin Taylor, Anne Koudokourmoff, Anthony Habert, Stacie Lewis, Danielle Littlejohn, Stuart Page, Neil Johnson, Matthew Docwra, CC Deville, Brett Widdows, Litsa Anthis, Joseph Low, Helene Seddon-Glass, Yana Dolin, Joanne Lusher, Paul Flaxman, Verity Leeson, Andrew Simpson and John Hucker.

Finally, I would like to thank all of the people struggling with the periodic ravages of depression who have been kind enough and brave enough to give their time in helping us to try to better understand mood disorders. This book is for them.

Contents

I: Depression

Chapter 1
What Is Depression?

'Depression is like being in a black hole with absolutely no emotion. Only the sufferers know just how difficult it is'. *A patient discussing their depression*[3]

There are a number of illnesses that we can experience over a lifetime that bring excruciating pain to the sufferer and, by proxy, to those around them. Indeed there are many different types of pain and it is common to find several illnesses sharing a number of pain symptoms. I believe that the pain that those with major depression can feel is unique and the feeling of descending toward that pain as another episode of depression begins is a fear unparalleled in the illness spectrum. Severe depression is an often relentless illness that strips sufferers bare of every tool they have to cope with everyday life until they can be reduced to an unrecognisable shell of their former self; feeling like a real person in name only. The above quote was taken from a patient with depression and is by no means unrepresentative of how many depressed patients feel at their lowest point. Depression can inhabit the sufferer and talk through them. It can live within like a parasite that takes control of sufferers' thoughts and feelings and make them feel like strangers in their own bodies. So how do we, as mental health professionals and the public, understand such a profoundly disabling and sometimes amorphous illness? I will begin with a few important facts about depression.

The WHO in combination with the World Bank noted that, in terms of years lived with disability, psychiatric illnesses were the most important contributors accounting for 30% of the total. Unipolar depression (that is, not including bipolar or 'manic depression') is responsible for 1% of deaths but 11% of the disease burden worldwide. In 1990, major depression, defined below, is the fourth highest source of disease disability and is projected to rise to number two by the year 2020.[4] Clearly depression is a serious health issue and one whose consequences are considered to be on the increase in the years to come. The sheer extent of despair and difficulty that sufferers and families experience is unique for a number of reasons but even today many fail to accord the condition its status as a serious illness. Before going on to discuss the way that depression is represented both by professionals, the media and the public, and indeed the importance of these representations in contributing to the difficulties and challenges experienced by sufferers, I will discuss the way that it is typically understood in Western medicine.

Major depression is significantly linked to suicide and it has been estimated that most of the 4000 people who commit suicide in the UK each year suffer from depression.[5] It can affect the long-term course of illnesses such as breast cancer, malignant melanoma and cardiovascular disease and has a significant cost to the workplace (although this is not often the primary concern of those in the midst of a disabling episode of depression) in absenteeism, reductions in productivity, medical visits and hospitalisation. Indeed the rate of working days lost is fourfold over non-depressed participants.[4] Between 50–85% of people who have an episode of depression will have a recurrent episode[6] and it tends to strongly co-occur with anxiety disorders (55%) and substance abuse (45%).[7] Since so many people with depression have multiple episodes and since each new episode tends to be more severe and occur more frequently, it is easy to see how the disease could seriously affect occupational status. Problems at work can very quickly become a symptom and cause of the disease if an unsympathetic manager takes it upon themselves to performance-manage a seemingly lazy malingerer out of their company. This is not uncommon and a poor understanding of the illness among the public can contribute to this lack of support.

Clinical Symptoms

There are two prominent international psychiatric diagnostic criteria, the International Classification of Diseases or ICD-10 and the Diagnostic and Statistical Manual of Mental Disorders or DSM-IV and, with regards to depression, these manuals share very similar definitions of depression. DSM-IV has split depression into major and minor depression, whereas ICD-10 uses mild, moderate and severe depression but many symptoms of the classifications overlap. The development of these criteria and the importance of the decisions made by health professionals to reify certain concepts related to depression are discussed in detail in later chapters but for now my discussion will be limited to what these definitions are and what they mean.

The DSM-IV criteria for an episode of major depression stipulates that the sufferer must experience five or more of a certain group of symptoms during the same 2-week period and that this must represent a change from previous functioning. At least one of these symptoms has to be depressed mood or a loss of interest or pleasure. The other symptoms include such areas as:

- Significant weight loss without dieting or weight gain
- Insomnia or hypersomnia (too little or too much sleep)
- Psychomotor agitation (a series of unintentional and purposeless motions. These include pacing around a room, wringing one's hands, pulling off clothing and putting it back on, etc.) or retardation nearly everyday (that can be observed by others rather than subjectively felt by the sufferer)
- Fatigue or loss of energy nearly every day
- Feelings of worthlessness and/or guilt

- A diminished ability to think or concentrate or indecisiveness
- Recurrent thoughts of death or an actual suicide attempt.

The designated differences between minor and major depression and between the ICD-10 categories of mild, moderate and severe depressions tends to be how many of these symptoms are present rather than representing a given qualitative clinical difference.

It should be noted that these symptoms should cause clinically significant distress and impairment to the patient's social and/or occupational functioning and not follow an experience of bereavement. A number of clinical instruments have been designed to allow health professionals to measure whether a given person meets these criteria for depression such that a diagnosis can be provided.

Now if the selection of five or more symptoms over a 2-week period appears to be arbitrary to the discerning reader then that is because, to an extent, they are. Through my own research I have seen a number of people who have shown three or four symptoms, including the cardinal symptoms of depressed mood and lack of interest, for a prolonged period of time or people who have over five symptoms for periods of a week to 10 days. Furthermore, such criteria represent static descriptions in symptomatology that tend not to describe the range of fluctuations that exist during the course of the illness.

One profound point of dissatisfaction for many is that the same term has been used for a clinical illness, a symptom or an everyday mood change and this has very likely contributed to the stigma felt by sufferers of depression over the years. If public perception holds that someone suffering from a critically disabling period of major depression is no different from someone feeling a bit 'down in the dumps' then sympathy may well be in short supply for the sufferer. In actual fact, the link between feeling a bit blue and depression is similar to the link between a 'scratch and a compound fracture'.[8] The importance of anhedonia, or the lack of a capacity to feel pleasure, is often paramount and depression has been understood (certainly by many sufferers) as a lack of vitality, a feeling of pure emptiness where a sufferer can feel no interest in any of the people and pursuits that previously engaged them. The opposite of depression is not necessarily happiness but vitality, being able to experience a full range of emotion, including happiness, excitement and sadness and this anhedonic emotional flatness can be one of the most agonizing aspects of the illness. Major depression is not an emotion. Sadness, disappointment and fear are emotions. Major depression is an illness and this perceived link between feeling down in the dumps and major depression is one reason that we find so many people with the attitude that sufferers of this incredibly painful and debilitating illness should just 'pull themselves together', as if such an action was within their capabilities (just like it was when the accuser might have felt disappointed or down in the dumps). The manageable dips in everyday life barely touch on the illness in its most insidious and catastrophic representation. Such an attitude is not likely to be prevalent in heart disease or diabetes but depression is a mental disease and they can be very difficult to perceive if you do not have personal experience of them. This is discussed in greater detail in Chap. 2.

Should It Be Depression or Depressions?

One of the principal points of contention in the literature over the years concerns whether depression is a unitary disease or a term that encompasses a number of diseases or types of depression. Depression is currently viewed as a single condition with a number of clinical variants, although some authors have argued for a categorical model that allows for different kinds of depression[9] or a more dimensional model. Terms such as endogenous and reactive depression have been used in the past and are still clinically useful according to some professionals. Reactive depression is depression that occurs as a reaction to some external event or groups of events whereas endogenous depression is believed to develop internally in the absence of these events, to represent a more biologically based change in events. Indeed feelings of loss and disappointment appear to be central features of most life events that precipitate depression.[10] After 80 years, we still entertain nebulous concepts of what represents 'reactivity' with regard to depression and it has been suggested that there is strong evidence that symptoms characteristic of endogenous depression cluster together to form a specific pattern.[10]

It has also been suggested that these differentiations are more useful for research than clinical purposes since pharmaceutical treatment is unlikely to be withheld on account of the sufferer being unable to explain a sufficient series of events to justify their depression. In short, the same treatment will often be issued regardless of the aetiology (cause), which tends to diminish the importance of the aetiology. Of course it is possible that the seemingly endogenous depressive may have an event that has precipitated their depression; they might just be unable or unwilling to recognize it. It is also possible for patients to suffer both reactive and endogenous depressions at different times in their lives.

The concepts of endogenous and reactive depressions make more sense in the context of the occasions and difficulties that may or may not precipitate depression. I have talked to many sufferers who report feeling perfectly happy and content before an episode of depression and many of these people have a tendency to choose to explain their illness as a biological and chemical imbalance as they can see no possible way that it was precipitated by external events. Some patients feel very strongly that they know what caused their depression and feel that the illness is a response to a given set of circumstances. Whether there is any qualitative difference with regard to the way that these different depressions are represented physiologically is debatable but that does not mean that the difference is clinically insignificant. Indeed the way that people cope with their disease, their treatment schedule recovery and other related aspects depends very much on how they understand its aetiology. As such, the differentiation is undoubtedly important.

As we discuss further in Chapter 5, a number of social, economic and political influences can play a role in influencing the aetiology and distribution of depression and to ignore these would be dangerously naïve. Losing a job, suffering bereavement, being exposed to an act of violence, a change in living environment, difficulties at work, financial strain or a long-term and disabling illness can, among other factors, play a profoundly important role in the development of an episode of depression. However, although these factors can influence the development of the illness, they do not have to be present for depression to develop. This is just one of the many contentious issues that contribute to our concepts of depression. Since little recourse is given to the possibility of different depressions, and the way that these operate, many overgeneralizations are made about the 'depressive' and the way that they behave. We may find people talking about all depressed people being perfectionists or being highly strung when, like most character-based generalizations, these are far from useful.

The group of symptoms above provide an impression of a very clinical and algorithmic process of differentiating the depressed from the non-depressed but they fail to express the excruciating psychological pain and apathy inherent in the disorder or indeed the havoc that it can wreak on sufferers and those close to them. They do, however, go some way to distancing the disorder from the vernacular representation of depression as 'feeling a little down'.

Dysthymic disorder is a related syndrome that falls within the depression 'family' and represents chronically depressed mood that occurs for most of the day, more days than not for at least 2 years but that does not reach the necessary number and duration of symptoms for major depression. Here, individuals often describe themselves as 'sad' or 'down in the dumps' but it is a chronic and long-term expression of symptoms. It is unclear for many clinicians whether dysthymia actually represents a disease distinct from major depression.

Depression and Cognitions

Depression is a disease that affects thoughts, emotions and the physical body, encompassing all aspects of the human experience, and cognitions (or thoughts) play an important role in the onset and maintenance of the disease. Since there are a number of theoretical schools in mental health, there are a number of different ways to construct the disease and the 'cognitive school' has been prominent in recent years. Some of the problems experienced during major depression include decreased lingual complexity, paucity of thought, reduced motivation, memory and concentration issues as well as a selective bias toward negative autobiographical events. Depression is often considered to be characterized by an 'inaccurate' cognitive style among other elements.[11] It is thought that many depressed people have negative cognitive styles, negative ways of thinking and retrieving knowledge and memories, and that these negative cognitive styles are associated with a more chronic course of depression. Self-blame and self-criticism are cognitions common to many depressives. This is also true of intrusive negative memories. Most depressed people experience highly specific intrusive memories concerning illness, death in the family, episodes of personal illness and assaults, relationship problems and rows.[11] It is thought that the onset of depression can trigger certain internal information-holding structures called schemas. These schemas represent specific information in the brain and it has been considered that the onset of depression could trigger a 'self-as-worthless' schema and this may then maintain the depression as the episode worsens.[11]

Prevalence

It is generally difficult to know the exact prevalence (number of people with the illness) and incidence (number of new cases of depression every year) of major depression. Due to the different methodologies, instruments and patient populations used to measure it and indeed to the different groups of countries and cultures represented in these figures, there has been quite a variety of estimates over recent years. Furthermore, problems with the use of different diagnostic classification systems mean that one of the few points of agreement is that the condition is increasing. The incidence rate tends to vary and has been estimated recently from as little as 0.07% in Swedish males[12] to 7.5% in Russia.[13] The 12-month prevalence of depression or number of existing cases varies widely from 3% to 15%, although some studies have suggested that specialized populations have prevalence's outside of this range.

In a recent study, a diagnostic interview was used to collect data from 15–54 year olds in the community in the US. Major depression and alcohol dependence were the most common psychiatric disorders and more than 17% of people had an episode of major depression in their lifetime, and 10% in the last 12 months. The major burden of psychiatric disorder is concentrated in a group of highly comorbid people who constitute 14% of the population.[14] Women suffer from depression considerably more than men and the general figures from different research suggest that there appears to be twice as many women than men with depression. Furthermore, the highest prevalence of depression tends to be in the 25 to 34-year-old group, declining with age.

So What Causes Depression?

Typical of a disease with no fully accepted aetiology, there are a number of psychological and biological theories of depression that have developed over the years. This chapter will not provide a comprehensive discussion of these factors, rather an overview to give the reader a taste of some of the principal theorizing that has explained the cause of depression. To fully understand these theories and their genesis requires a fuller understanding of both depression and the history of the mental health sciences, both of which are provided in later chapters.

In common with many other mental disorders, theories of the causality of mood disorders can be placed within psychological, social and biological perspectives. The psychological perspective traces the cause of mental disorders to past events, often remote to the sufferer, that impinge on current emotions and cognitions, whereas the social perspective tends to focus on the impact of interpersonal and social events external to the sufferer. These two perspectives tend to employ the mind–body dualism of Descartes and lean heavily on psychological constructs to explain the origin of depression.

The psychodynamic perspectives have traditionally focused on depression as the result of aggression or anger turned inward toward the self. This anger has been directed at a loved one who has thwarted the person's need for love and support. Because the person has internalized the love object in his attempt to prevent a traumatic loss, he becomes the target of his own anger.[15] However, this theory fails to provide an account of current forces outside of the individual, and recent developments in the psychoanalytic tradition have allowed a more active interchange between the mind and the environment. Adult losses, of which separations are the most frequent and potent, are postulated to revive a childhood loss and hence lead to psychopathology. This theory dovetails well with recent conceptualizations like the 'lock and key theory', discussed later.

Cognitive theories focus on the way people process information and became popular in the second half of the twentieth century. Prominent cognitive theories include those of Aaron Beck, a mental health professional who created the concept of the negative cognitive triad. Depressed people were said to have a negative view of the world, a negative view of themselves and a negative view of the future, and these people would commit 'cognitive errors or distortions' based on these three sets of beliefs. These errors are thought to maintain an outlook on life that perpetuates depression. Beck postulated that negative mental structures called schemas exist in a latent form and can act as predisposing factors to depression. Helplessness and hopelessness are seen as core experiences of depressed people.

Behavioural models of depression focus on the characteristics of people's immediate environment such as events of an interpersonal or situational nature. The theory of learned helplessness is one such theory. Based largely on animal experiments, the theory of learned helplessness states that a lack of assertiveness, passivity and resignation to fate are learned from the past where the person was unable to discover a behaviour that terminated aversive events. Thus helplessness is traced back to the personal biography of the patients.

Evolutionary theory is one strand of a more biological, reductionist approach to mental health and has also been used as a framework to explain depression (and, indeed, almost every other facet of human culture). Evolutionary theory states that depression is actually an evolutionary adaptation whose function is to inhibit aggressive behaviour to rivals and superiors when one does not have the resources to effectively challenge them. It acts as a kind of self-check mechanism to stop individuals competing and fighting for resources that they cannot realistically access and thus set up a dominance hierarchy without resorting to violence. Evidence from studies of primates has been used to support this view and humans are thought to share this yielding mechanism when competing for food or mates. It is self protective as it signals that the individual does not represent a threat. That said, while there may or may not be some merit in this explanation, I would have grave doubts about the success of evolutionary psychologists who try to explain to severely depressed patients that their current state serves as an adaptation. Just because a given illness is widespread within a species does not necessarily mean that it has an evolutionary origin. Heart disease and cancer are widespread but only the most extreme Malthusian group selectionists would ever claim either to be adaptive.

As with all psychological theories, each of the above conceptualisations have elements that feel intuitive when discussing some given aspect of depression but no theory alone is able to provide a completely convincing account of the full psychological, social and biological elements of the illness.

Children and Depression

Developmental factors have been assumed to create a vulnerability that disposes people to depression by either lowering the threshold to a wide range of triggering factors or, more selectively, triggers that have specific salience.[16] It has been suggested that the habitual experience of unpredictable and uncontrollable events can lead to learned helplessness. Research has suggested a link between childhood neglect, abuse and mood disorders and adult depression. Generally speaking, the more depressed mothers are, the less likely they are to be nurturant, affectionate and compliant with the child's dependency needs. They are also more likely to use physical punishment and harsh disciplinary procedures.[17]

It is thought that the sense of helplessness and unpredictability in children who are abused can lead to childhood depression. Students with a history of both psychological and physical abuse in childhood reported higher scores on the Beck's Depression Inventory, a commonly used questionnaire that measures current depression symptoms, than students who had not experienced these two types of abuse.[18] Furthermore, in a sample of UK women in the community, nearly all childhood forms of maltreatment were significantly related to lifetime chronic/recurrent major depression. Research has also shown that multiple abusive experiences are more predictive of outcomes such as depression than any one type of maltreatment. Furthermore, when assessing predictors of depression that lasts more than one year, childhood adversity in the form of parental indifference, family violence and abuse was critical. This is important since it infers that adversity can take a form other than what we might typically call 'abuse'. The category is thrown open to include parental indifference.

This work is particularly important because those patients with early onset tend to have a longer first episode of depression, sharply higher rates of occurrence, longer hospitalisation and greater lifetime substance abuse disorders. As such, misidentification when young is important and can lead to greater problems when older. While not being identified by general practitioners and other health professionals is a problem for adults and children with depression, adolescent misidentification tends to reflect diagnoses such as poor social adjustment, substance abuse and attention deficit/hyperactivity disorder, probably confounding the difficulties of these sufferers and their families.

From the interpersonal perspective, a number of unpredictable and uncontrollable circumstances are associated with developing depression. A sense of having been humiliated, a sense of loss (whether this is bereavement, loss of control at work and loss of status) and feelings of being trapped are often responsible for triggering episodes of depression. Such life events as separation and divorce from partners, long-term illness, psychiatric problems, disability, sexual and physical abuse, financial strain, alcohol and drug use, living environment problems and insecurity, relationship difficulties and problems at work have all been implicated. The way that these adult events relate to childhood vulnerabilities have been discussed by Parker and colleagues,[16] who suggest that there is a link between depressive 'locks' as a child and adult 'keys'. These could take the form of psychological vulnerabilities from childhood that were caused by physical or sexual abuse being triggered by adult events that elicited similar feelings, even though the stimulating event may appear to be completely unrelated. For instance prolonged physical illness with the associated feelings of reduced personal control, predictability and hopelessness may act as such a trigger. These 'locks' may not be related to keys in a logical and intuitive sense. Research showed that those rated positive for showing a lock and key relationship were younger and had been depressed longer. Furthermore, the links appeared to be stronger for those who were suffering with reactive rather than endogenous depression, although how much importance can be attached to this finding would be debated by many practitioners who believe that such a divide simply does not exist.

While this is interesting in theory, what we may be seeing, rather than a genuine lock and key relationship, is the adults interpreting the stressors and then applying that cognitive bias retrospectively and remembering and interpreting events in early life. This retrospective judgment is a problem with much of the research and theory that posits link between developmental issues and adult depression. Regardless, there seems to be enough evidence to implicate early experiences in the development of adult depression. The importance of this link and indeed what might be termed the 'generational aspect of depression', that of successive generations being at greater risk of developing the illness, is discussed in detail in Chapter 5.

Depression and Biology

As with all mental illnesses, biological explanations and implications have been eagerly sought from the scientific world. This includes drug companies seeking to effect a medication that would alleviate the symptoms of the condition, health professionals hoping to use their knowledge to better understand the biochemical basis of the illness or patient groups seeking to move the responsibility for the illness to biological complications beyond the patient's control. There has been too much dichotomy over recent years with regard to compartmentalizing aspects that are mental and those that are biological. Depression is, first and foremost, a biopsychosocial disorder and as such all three elements are crucial in its genesis, natural history and treatment. Mental illnesses have strong biological elements because fundamental elements of the experience of depression are represented using the biological apparatus inside the brain. Now the fact is that much of this apparatus and the way it works is still largely unknown to us in the early twenty-first century but what we do know is that the different constituents of the brain and the body are intimately linked. This is why depression is such a physical as well as mental disorder. Depression is represented not just by apathy, despair, hopelessness and sadness but by sleep difficulties, weight fluctuations, psychomotor retardation and somatic complaints. If it is possible to separate the way that the biology of mental illness has been used politically by interested groups (more of which in Chapter 6) and focus on the illness itself, the research paints an interesting picture.

A number of factors including stress, genetic predisposition, social networks and life experience interact to determine vulnerability to mood and the physiology of stress has received particular attention with regard to depression. The limbic brain is a command post that receives information from different parts of the body. It responds by regulating the body's physiological balance and maintaining homeostasis (internal biological stability). It essentially processes information in order to ensure our survival. When something stressful occurs, processes in the brain activate what is known as the hypothalamic pituitary axis (HPA). The hypothalamus, a constituent of this HPA, will act via the pituitary gland with the result that abnormally high levels of a stress hormone called cortisol is circulated around the body. This abnormal secretion can be beneficial in coping with immediate stressors but prolonged secretion can lead to problems with the immune system and depression. This endocrine arousal can be driven by feelings of chronic uncertainty and helplessness and the usually precise hypothalamic regulation of cortisol is impaired in many people with major depression. Indeed, high levels of cortisol are related to more severe depressions.[19]

Early social stress in non-human primates generally leads to disregulation of the HPA axis and this is also believed to be the case with humans. Exposure of the HPA to stress leads to decreased glucocorticoid receptor density in this hippocampus and the prefrontal cortex, an important area of the brain involved in planning and complex cognitive behaviours. This is possibly due to the chronic over secretion of cortisol and is important because decreased hippocampal volume has been found in major depression.[20] When you have relatively few receptors swamped by a great deal of cortisol you have a precursor for depressive illness. Regarding these lower hippocampal volumes in patients with major depression, studies suggest that this volume reduction may happen early in the course of depression or even precede the onset of the illness. Either smaller hippocampal volumes are a risk for depression or the atrophy occurs early in the course of the illness.

Specific early life stressors have been shown to be associated with HPA abnormalities. Women with child abuse histories showed elevated peak ACTH levels (a hormone involved in the physiological chain that leads to cortisol release), and childhood abuse (physical or sexual) is associated with smaller hippocampal volume. The effects of early damage to the brain may not appear until several years after the damage occurred.

Blood Flow

The amygdala (a subcortical structure in the brain that plays a special role in fear and is involved in the regulation of emotions and emotional memories) is the only structure in the brain that has been found to consistently show increased blood flow with depression. Its activity also correlates with cortisol levels. For recovered patients who have suffered from depression, the amygdala (particularly of the left limbic cortex) displays an increased blood flow compared to normal participants. As such, this site, where memories are stored and coded to feeling states, may represent a site for biological vulnerability.

Research has showed that comparing brain scans with depressed and non-depressed individuals show significant differences in blood flow in specific quarters of the brains, especially in the verbal and dominant left hemisphere. Decreased cerebral metabolism and cerebral blood flow have been reported in patients with a family history of depression.

Serotonin and Norepinephrine

There is a widely held view that depression involves a deficiency of neurotransmitters such as noradrenaline and serotonin in the brain. Drugs called selective serotonin reuptake inhibitors (SSRIs) block the reuptake of the neurotransmitter by the neurons or nerves in the brain that release it and so there will be more neurotransmitter in the neuronal synapse (the space between adjoining nerves). This results in other neurons in the brain being strongly simulated. Patients with major depressive disorder have low levels of norepinephrine and serotonin and so these have been implicated in the illness. It has been postulated that antidepressants exert their effect by reversing neuronal degeneration through the increased availability of neurotransmitters.

Genetics

The role of certain genes has also been explored in the recent medical literature, and a functional difference in a gene known as the 5 HTT gene was found to moderate the influence of stressful life events on depression. People with one variant of this gene showed more depressive symptoms, diagnosable depression and suicidal ideation in comparison to those with another variant. This has been taken as evidence for a gene/environment interaction where people with the more unhealthy gene variant will be more likely to develop depression in the presence of stressful or difficult life events.

The longitudinal relationship among childhood maltreatment, abuse and adult depression was also found to be significantly moderated by this gene. It should, however, be noted that this relationship between genetics, depression and environmental stress is still somewhat controversial and not all work in the area has found that this gene does actually produce a moderating effect between environmental stress and depression. At this stage it is best to be cautious when interpreting the results of these studies. Methodological differences often play a result in the variance in findings with results such as these.

To describe the cause of depression in singular terms can be a fairly empty pursuit as different people experience different causes for different episodes of depression. Indeed later chapters take a critical appraisal of the political and economic value of the explanations and constructs used by the psychological sciences to understand mental illness and depression. It seems better at this stage to draw general themes rather than try to achieve such specificity in our definitions. Authors and health professionals currently speculating on the causes and chain of events that lead to depression have tended to endorse biopsychosocial theories that incorporate a number of different interacting elements that are linked together like a chain. A series of perturbing events or dislocations to social routines such as some kind of valued loss, either real or perceived, overwhelms the regulatory systems and lead to exhaustion. Sleep rhythms become disturbed. The disruption may not be excessively disabling, much like a minor ailment but whether such a development leads to depression depends on a number of biological, social or psychological elements including a constitutional genetic predisposition. Such a predisposition may mean that a sufferer is affected more deeply by dislocations caused by life events. Interplay with genetically and developmentally vulnerable systems in the amygdala and other limbic regions can then lead to depression. Some people may be liable to self-blame and negative thinking, which can lead to a downward spiral where motivation may become disabled. Depressed patients often talk about how they feel that they are 'going under' and this process can feel inevitable and out of control. The person can often recognize this loss of control and it will lead to increased levels of distress until a fully blow episode of depression is encountered.

Such an explanation or group of explanations accounts for many experiences of depression and a consideration of post-partum depression makes particular sense within this context. The postpartum experience involves several challenges such as hormonal imbalance, high expectations, sleep and physical regulation, perceived or actual lack of support, lack of control, uncertainty and feelings of failure that could combine to affect the development of an episode of depression.

What Does Depression Actually Mean to Sufferers and Families?

Until now I have talked about depression as it is understood by clinicians, the way it might be represented in health and mental health texts. The true horror that the experience of depression can represent needs to be described in a more anecdotal fashion. Since the experience of the disease can be idiosyncratic and very different between different sufferers (and indeed different episodes that a given sufferer may experience can differ considerably), providing a defining impression of the disease is a difficult task. In some ways, it is easier to view individual experiences or 'depressions' apart but I hope to provide some idea of the depths of despair that the illness can produce.

'Melancholy persons are foreigners in their mother tongue. The dead language they speak foreshadows their suicide'. *Julia Kristeva*[21]

Florid descriptions of the agony that severe depressives feel abound in the recent literature.[8,15] As depression worsens, so can feelings of flatness and apathy. There is often a lack of ability to engage with the world and an incredible feeling of frustration and emptiness, so powerful as to be agonising. Depression has also been described as feeling hopeless and full of despair, a slower way of being dead. Some patients often describe it as 'like being in a black hole with absolutely no emotion'; that other people often 'don't understand the emptiness, the feeling of a vast nothing' and many sufferers feel that only they know just how difficult it is.

Depression can erode people's capacity to give and receive affection, to connect with others and frequently leaves the sufferer feeling isolated and abandoned. This feeling of isolation is common since the illness is so unique and so powerful that, for many, it is impossible to comprehend. But then unless you have experienced it, how could one be expected to understand all-consuming feelings of emptiness and hopelessness that render one powerless to lead a normal life. Imagining physical pain is not a profound stretch for many people since almost everyone has experienced it at some time in their life, even if only from something as routine as a toothache. To imagine mental agony is a different matter and many people feel that they do not have the resources to draw on in order to fully understand this.

Unlike with many somatic diseases, the very vessel that you use to communicate is affected by the disease. The symptoms are not separate from the communication of the symptoms and so this makes consultation and treatment such a challenge. Even explaining the illness and its symptoms can be a chore and a burden that depressives reject, leading to further isolation from family and friends. With recovery, depressed people can often find it difficult to fully recall the pain they were in, how they could suddenly care so little about the future, about their jobs and their families. If this is difficult for the recovered depressive then it will be even more so for loved ones who live through this cycle of illness and recovery together with the sufferer.

William Styron, the author of Sophie's Choice, refers to his depression as 'madness' since the word 'depression' is simply an inadequate expression for the experience and indeed since 15% of all the people with major depression will end their lives by suicide, the degree of suffering should never be underestimated. Depression can infest all of the normal behaviours and habits that constitute normal living and the thoughts of depressives can come to bear no relation to reality. Routine habits become neglected, planning becomes a difficult burden, thinking is slowed often to the point of the sufferer being unable to carry through thoughts, and concentration is scattered. What Whybrow[15] calls the 'housekeeping functions' can become completely unsynchronized. Sleep and appetite become disturbed with too much or too little of either. The episodes feel utterly crippling and the person comes to feel like a hostage to the disease. Indeed some live in fear of the next episode, expecting that any day soon they may descend into this maelstrom of madness, agonizing emptiness and churning despair. For many, a numbing preference for death emerges from the overwhelming sense of hopelessness that infests every part of their life.

The seeping feeling of numbness and apathy can render close family and loved ones as complete strangers and slowly, the many reasons that people have for living begin to evaporate. Not all depressives attempt suicide and indeed not all depressives even experience suicidal ideation but a great many do and death begins to formulate as the only escape available from this non-living that they are experiencing. When motivation and hope are taken from them, many fail to see the episodic nature of their distress; that it is a period of illness that will inevitably end and, when in the middle of an episode, many depressives report the feeling that the agony and emptiness will never end. Depression can take away hope for the future and hope for recovery so that there is nothing ahead. The belief in temporality is one of the most important protective factors and is often the first thing to go and the last to come back.

Depression is a disease of loneliness, even for those surrounded by love. The feeling of loneliness is often external to the strength of the social network. The more episodes of depression that a person experiences, the more episodes they are likely to experience and this is one reason why effective treatment for first or index episodes is so crucial. First time depressives often experience a sense of confusion, which feeds into the desperation of helplessly watching their life as they know it slip away. This novel and indescribable pain seems to come from nowhere and there are a number of responses to coping with the disease. These include denial, medicalization and desperately reaching for explanations and justifications for this new distress. To experience agony is one thing, to not know why or when it will stop or when it will start again can be unbearable and can add to the feeling of emotional inertia felt by many sufferers. A great many depressives have no idea why they become ill. One hundred and one intuitions are developed and tested when they have the motivation and wherewithal to do so but they usually fail to provide the answer. Moreover, nor do a great many health professionals in many cases.

Of course, the effects I have discussed are generalizations and every experience is, to a degree, idiosyncratic. Depending on their life story and their vulnerabilities, people will experience different types of depression but many of the themes overlap. However, the suffering one experienced during one episode can be very different to the distress of a new episode. Where before a person could be suicidal with great physical discomfort as regards agitation and anxiety, a second episode may be experienced as anhedonia and fatigue.

The Experience of Loved Ones

'I felt I had no friends and no future. I couldn't see more than 5 feet away'. *Andrew Solomon*[22]

As an inevitable result of some of the problems mentioned above, depression can tear into family structures with savage effect, leaving friends and relatives hoping and praying that this seemingly random and obstructive disease, of which few non-sufferers can truly understand, dissipates. To experience this from the outside and watch a close relative be swallowed into this seeming nothingness is extraordinarily painful and frustrating.

Relatives try to find solutions, lifestyle solutions, health solutions, medication solutions, anything that might help this person who is often no longer motivated to help themselves and there are few things as frustrating and painful as the feeling of fighting depression on your own when the sufferer has bailed out. This is an all too common feeling for many relatives. It is no-one's fault, just another debilitating symptom of the illness.

Many experience feelings of guilt when they temporarily break off from their depressed relative for a brief respite of social interaction, knowing that the depressive simply cannot experience that kind of pleasure and enjoyment. Depression is, by its very nature, a profoundly introspective illness, one of *the* most introspective. The nature of the internal pain, thoughts, memories and feelings and the inability to break from these for any prolonged period of time, means that the depressed person is so often enveloped in their own suffering. Having talked to relatives, it becomes obvious that one of the great problems is being unable to generate any kind of focus outside of the sufferer. They have to work hard to break the long periods of silence and introspection because many apathetic depressives will not voluntarily engage in conversation. Often the only break from these silences can be to discuss the illness, how the patient is feeling, what they would like, or how you can help, and so the choice soon becomes silence or depression for the close relative. Neither of these are particularly pleasurable for the relative; nor are the feelings of guilt, which accompany the realization that sometimes you want a break. Sometimes they do not want to talk about how bad the sufferer feels, how hopeless they feel and how they cannot see a way out. They just want a break.

Another issue can be the hurt caused by the realization that the sufferer has lost the ability to care about you and about their life with you. If they feel so hopeless and empty and care so little about everything then how does that impact upon the family member or friend? It can contribute to the difficulty associated with the role of helper and even though the family member knows that it is the illness 'speaking' rather than the sufferer, it can still take a great deal of empathy and patience to temporarily accept these circumstances while the patient suffers. Everybody needs a degree of positivity and validation from time to time and to receive so little from someone you care about and love so much can be devastating and utterly draining.

Children can also be profoundly affected by parental depression and can have a tendency to become 'pseudoadults', with the extra responsibility of an inverting of roles with the child often looking after a parent day after day. It is not uncommon for such children to act out later in life due to the anger they feel at being emotionally abandoned. Neither child nor parent are to blame for such a situation but it can be very difficult to remain unaffected when, as a ten year old, you are trying to get your parent out of bed when you come home from school.

Depression, Suicide and Substance Abuse

One of the key issues surrounding depression regards the issue of suicide and suicidal ideation. The concept of suicide means different things to different sufferers and can be used in different ways. Some depressed patients never consider suicide, some barely even reflect on death but for many, thoughts about death can be a part of their depressive experience. Many live in fear of their suicidal thoughts, scared that they will eventually lose the will to live and the ability to fight this illness that is dominating them.

Some sufferers can come to take comfort from the option that suicide presents. It can act as an unknown cure, an untried option just like drugs, alcohol and antidepressants; something that can be accessed when despair and panic are overwhelming. When in complete despair and emotional agony, when panic, desperation and fear become too great, the knowledge of a possible cure or 'way out' is knowledge of a possible respite.

Some patients, when rationalizing their illness at the early stages, try to halt the despair by convincing themselves that this episode is not as bad as previous episodes because they have yet to cross a given barrier (whatever that may be) that denotes a worsening of their condition. This may be taking medication or seeing a GP or telling someone close or staying home from work but they can become fearful of crossing certain boundaries as it removes a barrier to the acceptance that they are once again depressed and without hope. Knowing that this episode has not yet required you to take medication (and hence must be less debilitating than previous episodes) can be comforting.

Substance abuse can act in a similar way and a great deal of depressed patients self-medicate with alcohol and other substances and indeed one-third of all completed suicides are alcoholics. Substance abuse can begin as a defense against depression but can eventually contribute to causing depression. When the present and future is bleak, then little thought is often given to the harm caused by substances. This immediately becomes less important and in the ranking of the depressed person's imperatives, dehydration, headaches and even liver damage come a very poor second to the despair and hopelessness they feel when depressed.

So how important is suicide in the grand scheme of things? How many people do we know who have committed suicide or have been touched by the effects of suicide? Many people are surprised when they hear that in the US in 1997, more young people died of suicide than of aids, cancer, stroke, pneumonia, influenza, birth defects and heart disease combined.[22] Moreover, there are approximately sixteen suicide attempts for every successful suicide.[22] It should be noted that most depressed people do not actually commit suicide and hopelessness is a more prescient predictor of suicide than depression per se. One in five people with major depression will make a suicide attempt but an issue of semantics arises since so many depressed people are also hopeless. Of course, knowing that few depressed patients commit suicide is little comfort if a relative of yours is one of those who have.

Interesting conjecture regarding the mindset of suicidal patients has arisen in recent years regarding what is known as a 'state of cognitive deconstruction'. According to some researchers, suicide is characterized by a need to escape an aversive state of mind or situation and this is key. Aversive states of negative affect are thought to lead to a subjective shift to a cognitively deconstructed state. This involves less meaningful, less integrative forms of thought and low levels of awareness and thinking. The state is characterized by concrete, short-term thinking and there is a removal of higher meaning. Irrationality, risk-taking and disinhibition become acceptable and passivity increases. Extreme escape becomes a feasible option in such cognitive circumstances.[23] The extent that this applies to patients who are depressed is debatable but it forms an interesting perspective.

Lay Views on Depression

As much as any illness, depression has a very strong set of lay beliefs relating to different aspects of the illness. There are a number of reasons for this, more of which are discussed in the next chapter. However, not knowing the cause of the illness or when and why it strikes, in what can be a seemingly random, episodic fashion is important. Actual knowledge of what the symptoms are is also important since only 39% of the general public recognized vignettes from depressed people as being depressed.[24] Many sufferers do not themselves know what depression actually is and thus do not see themselves as unwell or they know the stigma that is associated with depression and can only see a negative outcome of associating themselves with such an illness.

Depression also violates the foundational work ethic so prominent in Western culture. Many view the illness as a failure in being self sufficient, in being able to cope with the normal vicissitudes of life and that those with depression lack an inherent strength with which to combat normal challenges. As such, sufferers are often tainted with inaccurate accusations of laziness or weakness, accusations that they may well level at themselves as they try to come to terms with the changes that they are experiencing. Indeed this self-recrimination can contribute to the downward spiral that they experience as their illness develops.

Nobody chooses to be depressed but many of the comments they face from others suggest differently. Being told to 'snap out of it' or 'pull yourself together' hold strong connotations of personal responsibility and one could be forgiven for thinking that such accusations reflect a belief that the sufferer has chosen depression for a little holiday away from their difficulties and responsibilities. I hope that through the course of this book, and particularly Chapter 2, the reader has been fully disavowed of such sentiments.

There are many misunderstandings and fears regarding the treatment used for depression and the patient's personal significance of his or her illness and their subjective experience of symptoms should be acknowledged properly. Accepting the use of antidepressants is, to many, accepting that they can no longer cope with the challenges of life without being pharmaceutically aided and sometimes a complete change of mindset about the disease will be necessary before fully accepting medication. Depression is an illness, much like epilepsy and diabetes are illnesses. As such, taking medication for depression should be considered a more natural and inevitable process than it is. Unfortunately, as is discussed in greater detail in Chapter 2, the stigma and connotations of personal responsibility associated with the disease means that asking some sufferers to adhere to medication can be a running battle.

Many patients cannot comprehend why you would take a medication or combination of drugs to address what they might see as insolvable social problems. Some believe that overworked GPs just over-prescribe antidepressants rather than help the patients to address the root cause of their problems and so many are skeptical about drug treatments but open to complimentary therapies. It is not uncommon to encounter the perception that health professionals write prescriptions too quickly and without actually taking time to understand the illness and, more importantly, the patient.

There is much debate about the suitability and effectiveness[25] of antidepressants as a treatment and this can tend to come from patients' perceptions of issues such as the likelihood that they will change their personalities or that the side effects will be insufferable. A fear of addiction is prominent, although nowadays the popular antidepressants tend to be less addictive than in previous years. Eighty percent of the population erroneously considers antidepressants to be addictive and 69% believe that their use would lead to personality change. Some GPs have noted that several consultations were necessary before patients' reluctance to use antidepressants was overcome.

In the UK, a majority of the public would be embarrassed about seeing a GP for depression.[24] Interviews and focus groups have suggested that depressed patients have a strong sense of people not being sympathetic to their problems[26] and a pervasive sense of being different and 'locked away'. Many regard their GPs to be too busy to deal with what they see as such a trivial issue. Unfortunately the disease itself can strip sufferer's self-worth to the extent that they may not see themselves as worthy of medical attention.

Recent studies of help-seeking preferences from the general public suggested that psychotherapy is the preferred treatment and it appears that the perceived role of family and friends has decreased together with an acceptance that proper medical help is necessary.[27] Most people feel that psychotherapy is a better first choice for depression than drug treatment. Psychotherapy is seen as addressing the real problems, the underlying issues where drug therapy simply covers the issues with a veritable drug-fuelled haze.

Such beliefs will have to continue to be addressed if we hope to improve the lives of many sufferers of depression. Indeed, as lay people become increasingly well-informed about health but maintain an acquiescent role in general practice then non-compliance with GP's suggestions for their depression treatment will continue to represent a problem.

Treatment for Depression

The number of prescriptions for anti-depressants in the UK went from 10.8 million in 1993 to 26.6 million in 2002. The issue of treatment for depression is a nebulous area for a number of reasons. Recovery for patients with depression is usually not straightforward or conventional, with setbacks a common occurrence. According to the WHO, after a single episode of depression the likelihood of another is 50%, after two episodes it increases to 70% and after three this increases to 90%.[9]

Not receiving treatment is associated with delayed remission of symptoms, greater functional impairment and an increased risk of suicide. Treatment decisions should generally be based on the type of depression, the severity of the illness, duration and history of the patient and their illness[28] with monitoring for pharmacological side effects and treatment compliance of crucial importance. Some health professionals feel that it is not necessarily the type of treatment that is important, rather the continuation of the treatment. This is especially important in a health culture that under-treats the illness. Moreover, taking account of patient preferences and their thoughts and feelings at the beginning of treatment is fundamentally important if we are going to expect the patient to continue with the treatment through what can be enormously challenging times.

The Statistics and Figures

The time has come to launch a barrage of statistics at the reader, for a full understanding of the issues surrounding treatment is not possible otherwise. Overall, less than 10% of patients receive adequate treatment for their depression and between 75 and 90% of patients will experience multiple episodes of the illness.[4] It is thought that with each new episode, subsequent episodes occur sooner and with greater severity than the previous episode and so treatment efficacy has very serious consequences.[4]

Many people come to treatment expecting that once they receive their treatment they will then become well again. This is not unreasonable as it is based on a lifetime of experience regarding illnesses and the way that they are treated but, as with a number of illnesses, the story with depression is less straightforward. Pharmacological treatment is often used to facilitate remission rather than curing a patient per se and half of the people who use antidepressants will experience an unsatisfactory outcome with the first antidepressant that they are prescribed and half of those prescribed will be prescribed at a lower dose than is recommended.[29] Antidepressant treatment tends to have three phases. These are the acute phase (6–8 weeks), continuation phase (4–9 months) and long-term maintenance. Twenty-five to 30% of patients discontinue treatment after 1 month and 40–50% discontinue treatment within 3 months,[29] which is prior to completion of the acute phase of treatment, the phase during which treatment is most necessary. Since it is recommended that most patients take a course of antidepressants for between four and nine months, it can be seen that this is a genuine health issue. Indeed only a quarter of patients taking antidepressant treatment receive follow-up care over the next 3 months, the time period during which so many will discontinue their medication[29] and this discontinued use is predictive of increased risk of recurrence and relapse. Reflecting on these statistics, 64% of depressives have indicated that they have unmet needs regarding their care[30] and so it is clear that the treatment process for people with depression is far from ideal.

So, bearing the above information in mind, exactly how long can people expect to be depressed? Although figures vary as a result of geography and the methodologies used to measure them, a reliable interview used in a household survey in the US suggested that the mean duration of episode was approximately 16–22 weeks.[14] Further research has shown that between 47% and 68% of outpatients had reached remission of depressive symptoms after a year[29,31] and that 12%–17% were persistently depressed.[29] After five years, a US study showed that 12% of participants had still not recovered and that there were decreasing rates of recovery as time passed.[32]

A summary of the results can be difficult to interpret as there can be quite wide variance in the results but, as mentioned, what is well accepted is that getting the right treatment as soon as possible, and staying with that treatment, is the most effective way of avoiding long-term depression. There are a number of factors that have been found to be predictive of longer episodes of depression and while the significance of these is discussed in Chapter 5, they include such domains as marital status, years of formal education, employment status, social disability, being female, stressful life events and emotional support from family and friends.

Consulting: Why Do So Few People Seek Medical Treatment?

In the USA in 1990, only 12% of individuals with a mental disorder had used formal health services in a year. This figure was 20% for Canada, 41% for Australia, 69% for the UK and 33.9% in the Netherlands.[33] To understand these figures, we have to understand the patient and practitioner influences on the mental health consultation. The attitudes of patients and their families to seeking medical treatment for depression is fundamental to a swifter resolution of the illness and, as mentioned above, several key issues stand in the way of successful consultation for mental illness in primary care. Problems at the practitioner/patient interface for depression contribute to poorer levels of recovery from the illness. In addition to the problems mentioned above, it is also common for patients to feel anxious about taking up their doctor's time and experience heightened feelings of time pressure and general low entitlement when consulting their general practitioner for depressive illness. There seems to be a general feeling that these health professionals should only be contacted in extremis and those that do consult often leave the surgery with many unasked questions regarding the way they feel.[34]

Some patients are concerned that they will represent themselves as an unfit parent. The public stigma around the disease or a lack of personal knowledge about their illness is also relevant to this profound under-use of services. Many depressed patients feel that there is little point in consulting a health professional in the first place since there is nothing that can be done for their depression. The sense of hopelessness that infuses their outlook can influence their views on treatment and it is an unfortunate effect of the disease that many of those who need help the most will not receive it since they believe themselves to be beyond care.

Some people may have difficulty in opening up to their practitioner or expressing their feelings coherently. Most people with experience of publicly funded primary care would not be foreign to the experience of feeling rushed in this environment or having an experience of being rushed in the past. An average consultation time of eight minutes does not maximize the possibility of recognition, especially when the patient factors mentioned earlier fail to aid recognition. This time issue has been implicated in up to half of the cases of hurried consultations and they are not conducive to the disclosure of intimate and sometimes embarrassing personal details.[35] While many health professionals will be prepared to spend longer with a depressed patient than they would with other consultations, this is not generally known by patients, who assume that GPs simply do not have the time and resources to cope with their problem. This is a reasonable supposition since much of their previous experience will consist of brief consultations that have felt like a race against the clock. Busy waiting rooms do not encourage this perception.

Hence the overall effect of the issues described above is that many people do not utilize primary care for their depression and those that do will only infrequently be recognized. This is unacceptable but does not result just from characteristics of the patient or the illness. It also happens because of the attitudes and knowledge of health professionals.

Health Practitioner Attitudes and Knowledge

Texts on depression can have a tendency to focus on the patient and minimize the importance of the other people involved in the depression experience and health professionals are one such group that have been relatively neglected. There are a number of problems on the health professional's side of the desk that also make depression a poorly addressed illness.

Many depressed patients (up to 50%) are not recognized by their general practitioners, first because depression and the associated somatic complaints can be a difficult illness to isolate, and second because many general practitioners have an insufficient grounding in mental illness. Some general practitioners do not feel able or experienced enough to provide depressed patients with the correct treatment approach and some simply do not have the time.[36] However, the quick recognition and treatment of symptoms is essential. Depression is an incredibly frustrating illness to treat because the relationship between treatment type, treatment adherence and remission is not straightforward. Some doctors have been known to show negative behaviours and appear visibly frustrated when the desired improvements are not made.[37] Already hyper-sensitive patients can pick up on these cues and the doctor–patient relationship can be irreparably damaged.

Recent work in the US suggests that one of the primary differences between psychiatrists and general practitioners was a lack of practitioner confidence[38] and very few GPs conform to clinical practice guidelines.[39] This lack of confidence is probably responsible for one of the most institutionalized medical errors of our time. A great many GPs perpetually under-prescribe antidepressant medications and fail to prescribe medication for the recommended period of time.[40,41] This failure to treat depressed patients correctly can lead to relapse and the development of chronic and recurrent depression, not to mention a waste of health funds. Furthermore, these poor prescription practices may influence patients to move away from the antidepressant treatment option if they erroneously think it inadequate.

Practitioner beliefs are essential with regard to the treatment prescribed with the 'low dosage' general practitioners more likely to believe in the efficacy of psychotherapy over medications.[42] They also tended to be less comfortable in managing the illness than their counterparts who prescribe doses at a higher and more appropriate level. In defense of general practitioners, there exists a number of differing guidelines for treatment that vary considerably in quality and consistency.[39] This does not aid clear and consistent treatment protocols and indeed many general practitioners are not happy about the recommendations and guidelines for depression, especially the seemingly arbitrary nature of the time period(s) used.[43]

Communication between patient and general practitioner is essential and this is especially the case for depressed patients. The best predictor of concordance with treatment is the extent to which patients can discuss treatment options and select those that best fit the context of their lives. Also, patients need to be systematically followed-up (and this often fails to happen) with a necessary change in focus to appreciate that depression is a chronic illness that should be monitored as such.

With regard to the demographics of the health professional, it has been shown that female general practitioners gave more time to their depressed patients than males and that their consultation contained more effective talk and partnership building. Greater patient satisfaction is also found with female doctors.[44]

Adherence to Treatment

One of the principal problems regarding antidepressant treatment is patient adherence to the recommended treatment regimen. Patients' beliefs and attitudes are probably an even greater cause of non-adherence than their experience and fear of side effects.[45]

Many patients do not feel well informed about their medication and it is not uncommon for them to take less than the prescribed amount or stop completely. There are a number of reasons for this and a poor understanding of the medication and its psychological effects, the feeling of losing self-control and self-sufficiency and the decision by many patients to terminate or reduce treatment when they themselves feel better all contribute. Uncertainty over their medication can lead patients to experiment by stopping their use and a greater awareness of the nature of peoples' feelings about antidepressants allows health professionals to engage in a more focused discussion with patients and hence increase adherence.

The nature of non-adherence is rarely an all-or-nothing phenomenon with evidence showing that partial adherence is very common with just under 50% of patients acknowledging some degree of non-adherence in the last 2 years and 32% reporting only partial adherence to their antidepressant regimen in the last month.[46] Those who were shown to be only partially adherent were more likely to deny the severity of their illness and have been shown to be more likely to perceive the stigma associated with the illness and with relying on medications to function in an everyday context.[46] Other problems fundamental to the illness, such as memory problems and concentration, also influence the ability of patients to adhere to their medication. Those in low paid jobs or who are unemployed are particularly likely not to adhere to their medication.[47]

The earlier an antidepressant is discontinued, the more likely relapse is to occur and premature discontinuation with antidepressant treatment has been shown to be associated with a 77% risk of relapse.[48] We need better clinician awareness of the sheer scope of non-adherence and a better understanding of the factors affecting non-adherence. Positive factors that can improve antidepressant adherence are the use of a monthly, mail-based educational intervention, good quality communication between the health care provider and the patient,[48] strong family cohesiveness and the positive attitudes of others in the community.[47]

Are Antidepressants the Most Effective Treatment for Depression?

Antidepressants are generally considered effective treatments for depression and for long-term and severe depression in particular.[29] A recent study concluded that antidepressants and psychotherapy were equally effective for outpatients with mild to moderate depression but suggested that antidepressants were more effective for more severe depression. However, this remains somewhat controversial and this finding is not unanimously accepted as some people have found no difference between antidepressants and psychotherapy for primary care patients with more severe depression. Some work has suggested that cognitive and behavioural treatments for severe depression has produced clinical outcomes for patients with severe depression that do not differ from those achieved by antidepressants[49] and the recommendation that antidepressants should be unanimously accepted as a first line treatment for moderate to severe depression has caused some consternation among health professionals. Indeed there have been differences found depending on which specific types of psychotherapy and antidepressants are used and how these react with patient preferences and so the conclusions drawn at the moment are tentative.

Recent guidelines[28] suggest that either a number of different psychotherapies or antidepressants are suitable as first line treatments for depression. Second line treatments, those provided when first line treatments have not been effective, tend to augment the treatment chosen with psychotherapy or medication or try a different medication depending on the severity of the depression. Third line treatments tend to involve referral to psychiatric care or a second opinion whilst continuing with antidepressant therapy, and we can see from this regime that both types of treatment are integral to the process of depression treatment. As is often the case, the arguments on treatments for depression have been constructed in such a way as to resemble the gunfight at the OK Corral, with antidepressants swinging their six shooter at one end of the town and psychotherapy on the other. While this dichotomy is understandable as special interest groups mobilize resources to push their expertize toward economic and scientific reward, it is actually an impractical distinction if we view the discussion from the point of view of maximizing the benefit to patients. To offer both treatments in conjunction is often the most effective way of addressing depression. Medication can be used to alleviate the symptoms, while psychotherapy has been used to address depressogenic issues that may be troubling patients. Indeed some work suggests that this is more preferred by patients to either approach alone.[50] Not every patient responds to either type of treatment and the key to successful treatment is to appreciate the needs, preferences, fears and beliefs of the patient and to ensure close follow-up in order to monitor adherence.

Constant Medication: This Must be a Bad Thing, Right?

Some practitioners believe that more than two lifetime episodes should incline a clinician towards lifelong medication.[22] This is a contentious point since many believe that the function of medication should be to make a patient well. There is no sure evidence that a given person will become depressed again following treatment and so this could form an unnecessary intervention. However, my belief is that, if a patient has had a number of severe and debilitating periods of depression and an effective medication has been found to give them a constant and improved quality of life, then lifelong or prolonged long-term treatment is justified. We know that the more episodes a person has, the more they are likely to have to endure further and more severe episodes in the future and in this case the probable suffering and agony and possible threat to life is such that we can be justified in taking a perspective similar to that of long-term chronic medical conditions such as epilepsy and diabetes, where lifelong medication is often standard.

However, this issue is not straightforward. The constant use of medication for some can be a reminder of frailty, lack of strength and of a lack of independence but those with recurring and severe episodes of major depression would likely benefit. It is possible that for some patients, some time needs to be taken to help them through the transition that will allow them to take long-term medication without them viewing it as an inherent character weakness. Diabetes or hypertension would not be treated with a single medication treatment and nor should many experiences of depression. Further debate and a considerable re-education programme for physicians and the public would be needed before an adequate consensus is reached, which will maximize the benefits of medication for those with particularly severe and recurrent depression.

So What Do You Do if Medication Does Not Help?

Approximately 30% of patients do not respond to the usual recommended does of antidepressants and there appears to be a striking lack of guidance for medical practitioners as regards those with treatment-resistant depression.[51] There is considerable variance with regard to the different choices of treatment augmentation such as Lithium Sulphate, Tricyclic or MOA inhibitor antidepressants. In some countries, the most popular choice is to increase the dose or change the class of drugs rather than augment the treatment with another drug.[51] Any conclusion of the literature on antidepressants must acknowledge that, as a result of patient preferences and fears, general practitioner dispensing practices and variable recommendation and treatment guidelines, further work is necessary on the public health policy side of the equation. This will address structural issues that may be reducing patients' opportunities to benefit maximally from the pharmacotherapy available.

Beyond Drugs and Psychotherapy: Other Treatments
for Depression

A treatment that has been found to be useful with some cases of mental health issues has been Eye Movement Desensitization and Reprocessing (EMDR), a procedure where patients attend to past and present experiences in brief sequential doses as they simultaneously focus on an external stimulus or object. EMDR assumes that a trauma memory is information about an event that has been locked in the nervous system in almost its original form. The images, thoughts, sounds, emotions and physical sensations about the self (such as 'I am weak') are all stored together in a neural network in the brain that 'takes on its own life'. EMDR evokes this memory and all the associated emotional and cognitive components. By following the therapist's instructions with the appropriate eye movements, the process is thought to stimulate an innate information-processing system that has not been previously effective in healthily processing the dysfunctional memory. Dysfunctionally stored information is processed and the memory loses its power to create difficult emotions.[52] This theory is speculative although the results certainly seem positive and EMDR is a tool that could be useful where negative autobiographical memories play a prominent role in the depression.

Another form of effective treatment but one that has a very poor reputation is Electroconvulsive Therapy (ECT). ECT, partly as a result of representations in films and the media, has been stigmatized as a brutal and barbaric form of torture that harks back to former times when bizarre and painful treatments dominated mental health. Those who actually experience and view ECT are usually surprised by how clinical and modern the technique is and how much it differs from their previous perceptions. It is now a very smooth and simple treatment and ECT has been shown to provide marked improvement for 90% of patients. It is particularly effective for the very severely depressed and suicidal.

Alternative therapies are often used by patients with depression who do not trust, or feel they have been let down by, conventional medical approaches. St. John's Wort is one of the most prominent of these and although there is a plentiful supply of advocates for this treatment, there are also numerous critics who point to the lack of recognized research that has tested its efficacy. While St. John's Wort may well be useful for depressive illnesses, it is worth mentioning that the use of such substances often reflects a political ethos rather than decisions made with regard to medical evidence. St. John's Wort, like many alternative treatments, is attractive in a conservative and nostalgic way. It represents a return to a 'natural' way of treating illness and before modern synthetic creations distorted the process of treating diseases and these substances often have a particularly middle-class support base. This conservative perspective suggests that the means of treating illness in the past are, by definition, more trustworthy and effective as they are more natural and organic processes. The belief often holds that modernity has complicated the issue with vested interests creating toxic substances that benefit corporations first and patients' a distant second.

The bottom line is that people are allowed to choose whatever medications they wish for their depressive illness and usually have very good reasons for doing so. It is regrettable, however, when people do not allow themselves to experience modern medication that may alleviate their illness effectively and minimize the severity of future episodes as a result of misinformation or political perspectives that do not hold up under close inspection. Major depression should be treated as quickly as possible and unintentional ignorance over the benefits of natural products can interfere with this process.

Concluding Remarks

Capturing the essence of major depression is an activity fraught with difficulty and speaking about depression in general terms is not necessarily a useful approach. Depression can be a chronic long-term illness and it can exist as short recurrent bouts; people can have one episode of depression and never experience it again whilst others will be haunted by the disease throughout their lives, feeling that they exist in a terminal state of physical and emotional decline. Some may feel that they have no reason whatsoever to feel depressed and indeed, speaking objectively, they may not have. This might mean that they are more likely to consider their illness to be a chemical imbalance as opposed to a psychological reaction to events in their life. Alternatively, some may know, or think they know, why they are depressed and feel that a certain course of action will alleviate their suffering. Some depressives may experience incredible flatness of mood, apathy and a lack of interest whilst other may have depressed mood and sadness but have as much interest in their life as before their recent episode began. It is possible that some sufferers feel utterly hopeless and suicidal whereas the experience of another person may be particularly somatic in nature with fluctuations in appetite and weight as well as with their sleeping patterns. For some, it may come following bereavement and for others as a result of an illness. Some believe that a loss of control and power over the everyday events in their lives precipitated their depression and some, many, will have absolutely no idea why they are suffering as they are.

People with major depression may have all of the above symptoms or different symptoms with different episodes of the illness. Depression can be thought of as a phenomenon with symptoms that may wax and wane until, for reasons not yet totally understood, they cross a threshold at which point the person's condition becomes a major depressive disorder. It is, quite simply, an extraordinarily difficult concept to measure and standardize and we are still some way from a coherent understanding of the biological, psychological and social factors that interact to create the disease. Thanks to the formulations of the sufferers themselves, and generations of research, we have some pieces of the jigsaw but we are long way from the complete picture.

There are, however, a number of things that can be said about depression. Clinical depression is not simply 'feeling a bit down in the dumps'. It is a severe illness that can, and often does, wreck the lives of the sufferers and their families. The beliefs of sufferers, health professionals and society in general play a major role in influencing whether the disease is recognized and effectively treated and it is from this point that we carry the story to the next level. To fully understand depression and mental disorders generally requires an understanding of the history of medicine and a study of western modernity itself. Concepts of illness, especially mental illness, are very closely tied to broader social and political trends in society and to ignore these is to continue to perpetuate the treatment and recognition problems that so disable our approach to helping sufferers.

Why was the arbitrary diagnosis of depression decided upon? Where did this definition come from and what effect has this had? Why is there such great stigma surrounding the disease and how does this connect with the western tradition of individualism, personal responsibility and the work ethic? Why do so many people feel that the illness is akin to laziness or a flawed personality? The next chapter seeks to understand the way that depression is represented politically and socially in order to address these fundamental questions.

Chapter 2
The Stigma of Depression: History and Context

'I'd love to lie about it – invent an acceptable cancer that recurs and vanishes, that people could understand – that wouldn't make them frightened and uncomfortable'.[22]

For many people with depression, feelings of personal stigma are so pervasive that they are an inherent part of the experience and to tell another person that you are suffering from depression carries the fear of evoking feelings in others that range from confusion to distrust and disgust. For many, depression is quite simply not an illness and many fail to understand why others cannot just 'pull themselves together' or 'snap out of it'. For my own part, this makes about as much sense as telling a diabetic to snap out of a diabetic coma or telling en epileptic to snap out of his fit. Hardly appropriate behaviour but many people close to depressives tell them exactly this. Because of centuries of failing to understand the illness and a social and political perspective that has ran counter to the development of empathy for people with mood disorders, feelings of embarrassment, shame and self-disgust are rife within sufferers.

The link between mental illness and stigma is well established and this chapter discusses how these perceptions of stigma are borne and why they are so prevalent for sufferers today. To understand this, we have to better understand the history of depression over the centuries and the way that this history of depression has interacted with a history of individualism and personal responsibility. The difficulty in separating the self from the illness is a recurring confusion in depression and this lies at the root of much of the stigma associated with the illness. Unlike physical illness, you are the disease. When depression takes hold, it infuses every aspect of the sufferer's being and many have reported feeling disconnected, unable to recognize the person that they have become. Depression inhabits the sufferer and talks through them. It can live within and take control of sufferers' thoughts and feelings, often making them feel like strangers in their own bodies. As such, the judgment of others is not on some temporary, disembodied concept afflicting the body but of the sufferer themselves. They are unlikely to see physical symptoms like cuts or scars, bandages or a limp; they simply see the person, physically speaking, much as they did before. For this reason the sufferer is judged and not the disease.

The culturally entrenched Western beliefs regarding personal freedom and personal responsibility operate so that the depressed patients can be seen to be somehow 'allowing' this illness to engulf them. For many people depression and mental ill-health fall into the arena of the moral rather than the medical and losing control over the body as one might experience in a number of more physical illnesses is very different from losing control over one's thoughts and feelings. For a number of reasons, society chooses to sanction sympathy for the former but not for the latter.

A Brief History of Despair: The Journey from Melancholy to Depression

Ancient Greece

Reading some recent texts, one could be forgiven for thinking that depression and concepts of depression did not exist before the 1950s, the dawn of the antidepressant era, but a careful look at the literature suggests that concepts of depression existed in ancient Greece. Hippocrates, who played such an important role in the development of modern medicine, suggested that an imbalance in the four humours and an excess of black bile predisposed people to melancholy and he believed that such an imbalance could be induced by trauma. Black bile was also felt to be responsible for the 'demonic diseases' like epilepsy, dysentery and eruptions on the skin. Although the theory of the four humours and their effects on health failed to survive the transition to modern times, the generic concepts are still popular in some contexts, especially in the food industry where concepts of internal balance are claimed to be regulated by a number of modern wonder foods.

Plato was responsible for the revolution in thinking that posited a man's childhood as an influence on his character as an adult and he felt that the family environment was crucially important in matters of illness. Although these concepts were advanced for the world they lived in, the solutions for people who suffered from depression in ancient Greece appear to be anything but. In the post-Hippocratic world, some believed that placing lead helmets over the heads of depressed patients would allow them to be fully aware of their heads as they often complained of feeling 'light-headed'. As has been the case throughout much of history, explanations of a sexual nature were posited, with Philagrius suggesting that depressive symptoms emanated from a loss of excess sperm in dreams and believed that ginger and honey were the solution to the dilemma. Exactly how this might have explained female depression is less clear. During these times, sexual concepts were rife and some physicians blamed depression on an absence of sex, with many depressed patients being sent to their bedrooms. Since a lack of interest in sex is one of the features of depression, this solution probably felt particularly ungratifying for many sufferers.

A discussion of ancient Greece would not be adequate without a mention of the perceived role of the gods in generating mental illness. It was believed by many that mental illness was a direct punishment from the gods for previous misdeeds and in early Christian times was said to be a test of the faithful (which many, presumably, failed), sent by the devil. Aristotle believed that melancholy was less an illness than the natural temperament of the creative artist, a view that became popular again in early modern times.

The Dark and Middle Ages

During the early dark ages, physicians had begun to develop a different set of procedures to address melancholy in their patients. Rufus of Ephesus believed that the key was to reach the illness before it became established and that such activities as bloodletting, regular walking and travel would do just this. Other physicians used a range of 'treatments' to address the problem of melancholy. These ranged from the more benign, such as consuming moist foods and breast milk or placing the sufferer in a hammock, to punishing the sufferer, perhaps by placing them in chains.

Galen, the personal physician to Marcus Aurelius, became one of the most influential physicians of his age. He noted that his patients tended to experience interrupted sleep, palpitations, vertigo, anxiety, sadness, diffidence (symptoms that exist in the classification of depression today) and beliefs of being hated by God and/or being possessed by demons. Not for the last time medicine took recourse in a sexual genesis of symptoms, with deficient sexual release being the precursor for these brutal consequences. One patient has been reported as having being cured by manual stimulation of the vagina and clitoris after 'much liquid came out'.[53] Galen was also prone to developing his own recipes and potions to address the needs of this patient group and this reflected his predisposition towards psychobiological explanations for melancholy.

During the dark ages, St. Augustine declared that it was reason that defined men from the beasts and so a loss of reason was, by definition, a mark of God's disfavour. It was seen as a punishment for a soul that had sinned. Melancholy was a noxious complaint and represented a turn from all that was holy and sacred. Those who showed melancholy were not suffused with the glory of God's love. Worse than this, a deep depression was viewed as a sure sign of possession and melancholics were considered to be Judas-like in their treachery towards all that was holy. As a result, it was not uncommon for melancholics to be sent out to work under the presumption that this would cure them of their sloth and rejection of God's love. In the fifth century, Cassian, a monk and ascetic writer from Gaul, recommended that the brethren of the melancholic abandon him or her lest they too be guilty of a rejection of God's glory.

Alas this was not the worst treatment that was to befall the depressives. By the time of the inquisition in the thirteenth century, many were actually fined and imprisoned for their sin. St. Thomas Aquinas, a hugely influential theologian, doctor and philosopher, placed the soul hierarchically above the body and believed that the soul could not be subject to bodily illness. An illness had to either be of the body or of the soul and melancholy was assigned to the soul. During these times, the gift of reason was thought necessary for man to choose virtue, without it he could but sin against God. The soul was a divine gift and to feel melancholy was to sin against God directly. The medieval church henceforth defined the deadly sin of 'acedia' or sloth as particularly important. This word was common at the time and essentially described the symptoms of the melancholic/depressive. Unfortunately for melancholics, the most passionate clerics equated acedia with original sin and nominated acedia and idleness as the root of all evil. Hildegard of Bingen, a prominent writer and theologian, even went so far as to claim that Adam had melancholy coagulate in his blood the moment he disobeyed God's will.[53] As such, there was a drawing together of physical and mystico-religious symbolism, which acted to stigmatize melancholics with one of the great historical acts of defying God. If this was God's punishment to Adam, who had so sinned against him, then surely it was a punishment for the sins of the modern melancholics.

Disorders of the mind were particularly threatening during these times and explanations that postulated personal responsibility and deserving punishment placated a populous who lived in fear that they themselves might suffer such a curse. It also helped to ensure that the people thought twice about committing even minor religious transgressions lest they themselves develop this feared melancholy.

Modernity

As we will see in more modern times, concepts of mental illness and melancholy, particularly, have shifted through the ages. In direct contradiction to the dark ages and the middle ages, the renaissance glamorized melancholy as it came to be understood as a prerequisite to artistic inspiration and creation. The irrational pain and original sin of the middle ages was now beginning to be viewed as an illness. For Marsilio Ficino, one of the fathers of the renaissance and a profound influence on some of its most important writers and artists, this melancholy mind was now closer to God than that of others since it represented the inadequacy of its knowledge of God and was tortured as a direct result. It should be noted that not all concepts of melancholy changed equally in different countries and cultures but illness was gradually overtaking possession as the framework through which melancholy was explained. For instance in England, the illness grew to be associated with the aristocracy since those with the resources to travel to Italy and become inspired by the ideas of Ficino came back with this melancholic sophistication.[53] Everything had changed and melancholy represented sophistication, intellect and creativity and mock melancholy became the latest fashion accessory of the rich. This new enlightenment had not captured the church in the same way as it had captured the aristocracy and the sixteenth century saw the church forbid suicide to the extent that the family of the deceased would be punished by being stripped of all economic assets and possessions.

The end of the feudal system ushered in the era of modernity and the age of reason with a steady growth in market capitalism. Empiricist philosophers like Descartes and Locke questioned the role of church in society and the material world came to be understood only by scientific exercise rather than through reverence to the church. For the depressives who lived through these times, such a change in perspective may have been easier to accept than for the non-depressed since it could have been understandable to question what kind of benevolent God would strike them with such an agonising disease and then let society torture and humiliate them as a means of addressing it. Indeed in 1773, the poet William Cowper, due to his feeling of 'living in a fleshy tomb, buried above ground', was 'plunged into a melancholy and considered himself deserted by God'.[8]

Now that the tenets of science could explain and quantify that which had previously not been understood in the exterior material world, there was a movement towards locating the unknowable within the interior of the self-contained individual and this shift in perspective opened up a new front for this burgeoning science to attempt to quantify and comprehend. For some, this breakdown in the acceptance of a supreme and benevolent God led to a sense of existential alienation and confusion as the previous regime that had dictated and inspired their existence was rapidly changing. This revolution in thought was the new path to enlightenment and power was moving from the church to secular institutions. Depressed patients might have had little reason to fear such a change since religious hegemony had conspicuously failed to provide little more than hardship and brutality.

Although great scientific advances were made, this was not always reflected in societies' attitudes to the mentally ill. With the movement of the unknowable to the interior of the self-contained individual, mental health came to represent an aspect of self-discipline and so the melancholic would often be viewed as a somewhat self-indulgent figure rather than someone possessed of demons. Squalor and torture tended to be the experience of the mentally ill at this point with Boerhaave taking the time to suggest that patients be caused great physical pain as a way of distracting them from their mental anguish. As such, taking depressives to the point of drowning and regular torture was commonplace. As a result, many depressives understandably became reclusive and certainly circumspect on the topic of their suffering.

Following the initiation of the age of reason, the romantic period was once again a more understanding era for the depressive to live in. Kierkegaard and Hegel provided a philosophical platform for the acceptance of depression where people were exhorted to understand that 'any man with real intelligence will recognize the wretchedness of this condition'.[54] This era in the nineteenth century represented an element of rehumanization of depression and the mentally ill and a change in perspective that began to vitiate the torturous treatment of these people, so often forced into hiding.

With regard to aetiology, this new scientific approach was providing discoveries that lent themselves to reinterpretations of what caused and constituted the illness. By the seventeenth century, Harvey's discovery of the circulation of the blood led to theories[8] based on faulty circulation which then in turn gave way to theories implicating the electrical properties of the brain.

The Nineteenth Century

With the nineteenth century came great industrial, social, political and medical innovations in both Europe and North America. In North America, the 'great awakening' involved population expansion and growing opportunities for commercial ventures for the colonists, originally hailing from Europe.[54] However, to maximize many of these potential opportunities provided by the unique and fertile land, a change in social and political outlook was required by the colonists and only the rapacious could maximally benefit from the new found opportunities. A movement from a communal ethic, which had existed in Europe for hundreds of years, to a more individualistic, separate and entrepreneurial ethos provided just such a way of making the most of these territories. Many communities were already infused with the work ethic of Protestantism. A reinterpretation of the word of God, already nebulous in these times of secular growth, contended that he wanted his flock to fend for themselves, to take the initiative and acquire material possessions and maximally exploit their environment.[54] Indeed, to not do so was to fail to embrace this new concept of God's glory and urbanization and industrialization combined with secularism to promote a growing sense of disorientation in many of the communities in North America. This confusion and isolation was not helped by the ravages of the civil war and concepts of shared understandings became severely strained in the new territories.

On both sides of the Atlantic, the era of the Victorians represented the peak of enlightenment thinking, this unstoppable faith in progress through science and profit and individual entrepreneurial application. Like North America, Europe was in the thrall of rampant capitalism, although a great history of community and communal living meant that adapting to the whims of individualism and capitalism has been a less straightforward process over the years. However, the enormous disruptions brought about by the industrial revolution led to a destruction of community life, immigration to the cities and unreliable employment for many. Many of the poor came to experience anxiety, confusion and hopelessness during these times and the only solution for many of these displaced wretches was the savagery of the Victorian poorhouses.

During the Victorian era, the devil had been well and truly discredited as the source of mental illness and, in keeping with the spirit of the times, mental illness became a failure of rationality and a failure of will. Early asylums focused less on treatment than on coercing inmates into complying with the rules of modern society. Practices such as restraint, imprisonment, vomiting, beatings, public humiliation, bloodletting and torture were the tools of choice.

By the mid-nineteenth century, the medical profession had wrested complete control of these asylums, although this did not automatically bring about improvements in 'treatment'. A new series of conditions like the vapors, neurasthenia and hysteria were popularized and tended to be used for middle and upper class patients who experienced a period of mental distress. Labels for mental illness continued to evolve; the patient who had convulsive cries and fainting spells in the eighteenth century and hysterical paralysis in the nineteenth century could today be diagnosed with depression or chronic fatigue.

The ability to express symptoms of depression had always been a difficulty for people in the years leading up to the Victorian era because of the religious outcry and inevitable social or physical punishment that would result. During the Victorian era, women particularly suffered with regard to the consequences of expressing their mental distress. As a result of their powerlessness, women suffered most from the whims of medical nomenclature as physical aetiologies were used to describe their 'mental weaknesses'. Today one might reflect on their lack of legal and political standing, their total economic reliance on men, or the multitude of patriarchal mores that governed their dress, speech and behaviour as possible causal factors in their mental travails. Victorian women were not allowed to express a number of unbecoming behaviours and anger, and depressive symptoms were included in this. As such, many of their symptoms showed up as somatic complaints that were considered to be acceptable during these times. This would then reinforce a culture that viewed them as naturally and inherently physically weak and vulnerable, imprisoned by the caprice of their reproductive organs; supposedly irrational and unpredictable in nature at a time when these were cardinal sins.

As the medical revolution continued apace, old school physicians failed to see why a medical man would have need of a microscope since diseases so obviously involved the whole person. To focus on tiny cells would have appeared senseless and counter-intuitive to many. However, this changed towards the end of the nineteenth century as Lister, Pasteur and Koch generated succeeding revelations regarding the role of microorganisms in disease. At this point, mental illness was undergoing a fundamental evolution itself and the arrival of Emile Kraeplin profoundly affected the way we would come to understand it in the following century. He suggested that mental disorders be split into two categories; those of manic depressive insanity and dementia praecox. These divisions essentially corresponded to the mood disorders and the schizoaffective spectrum of disorders.[53] Sigmund Freud was also rising to prominence at this time following his assertion that hysteria was caused by childhood sexual abuse, a claim he later retracted and restated.

Early Twentieth Century

The early twentieth century ushered in the widespread acceptance of psychoanalysis and psychodynamic theory. Freud had traveled to the US to lecture and the mental hygiene movement was founded, although the Emmanuel movement, containing many important advocates from the ranks of professional medical men, was still prominent with regard to maintaining the age-old link between religion and medicine. The psychological trauma experienced by soldiers in the aftermath of World War I helped to alter this.

The nineteenth century had seen the development of unfettered capitalism and laissez faire market fundamentalism. New societies were created in the UK and the US, and the ethos of communal living had receded into the distant past. This was driven principally by a wealthy political and industrial elite keen to maximize profits but with little regard to the quality of life of their workers/electorate. The brutality of World War I destroyed many of these concepts of laissez faire logic in Europe and a fundamental change in values was driven by the devastation of the war. Social democracy, political and industrial legislature, union representation and social service grew in Europe, a movement not reflected in the US where the devastation of the war had not affected them with quite the same force. In Europe, the moral and political compass was changing but in the US there was a general apathy towards such democratic staples as the antitrust laws. Child labor and violent union-busting tactics were dominant, although Roosevelt was prompted towards a degree of social democracy following the depression with the development of the New Deal.

At the beginning of the twentieth century, mental disorders were still well within the medical domain and restricted to a very small number. Such pioneers as Freud were keen to expand their professional domain by encouraging the relocation of psychiatric practice from the asylum to the office so that mental health professionals could address serious mental issues and also lifestyle issues, personal problems, unhappiness and deviant behaviour.[55]

The psychoanalytic movement and dynamic therapy, its treatment of choice, helped to draw together and cement the relationship between neurotic behaviour and normal behaviour so that both were considered different expressions of common developmental processes. This allowed professionals to potentially address anybody, regardless of their problem. Ordinary behaviour was argued to stem from the same origins as pathological behaviour, a focus removed from the more biologically based psychiatry that is currently in vogue. Dynamic psychiatry promoted the belief that by turning inwards and reflecting on their own histories, people could find the answers to their everyday ailments and serious psychological disorders. Social and political perspectives were sidelined in the haste to trace the origin of people's problems in events in their distant past and a growing group of psychodynamic analysts were prepared to support this.

The movement was initially popular with intellectuals and bohemians whose individual experiences prompted them to embrace individualistic solutions to their lifestyle dilemmas. This therapeutic movement was bound to flourish in the US, an individualistic culture that encouraged personal responsibility and personal freedom of choice. By focusing on individual historical biographies in such a narrow and intense manner, the movement synchronized perfectly with the prevailing cultural ethos of the US. It was a fundamentally conservative movement at heart, overcoming the repressive nature of social and community ties by providing personal solutions.

As with the experience of shell shock in World War I, the psychiatric experiences of World War II further emphasized the understanding that noxious environments can play a role in the development of mental disorders.[56] This new psychosocial framework acknowledged that the boundaries between those who are well and those with mental disorders is fluid and that these illnesses are continuous rather than discrete. The belief developed that anyone placed in a sufficiently difficult environment, whatever that may be, would be at risk of developing mental disorders.

American psychiatry continued to apply the psychodynamic and psychosocial model of mental illness to a wide variety of social practices like child rearing, junior education, business and poverty. It became a social panacea for those who were dissatisfied with their lifestyles, with their careers, their partners or their lives in general and a framework for a broad approach to modern psychotherapy had been established.

Psychiatric Classification

In the early 1950s, the development of the tricyclic antidepressants led to the evolution of measurement scales such as the Hamilton rating scale for depression, which became the gold standard measurement of current depression. At this point, endogenous depression was considered to develop from constitutional or genetic factors as it appeared to arise without any psychological or social precursors. It was this specific type of depression that such antidepressants and treatments like ECT were developed to address. Neurotic or reactive depression, which stemmed from life adversity, was considered to be more appropriately managed by psychoanalysis. The path to the development of a rating system based on a standardized instrument was not straightforward since many clinicians were unable to appreciate the utility of standardized scores for depression; that is, an aggregate of symptoms that could provide a measure of degree of disability. For instance, could the symptom of early morning waking or low appetite be considered equal to that of suicidal ideation or anhedonia?

Many clinicians remained skeptical about this instrument and other instruments like Beck's depression inventory, which they felt were overly individualistic with large areas of personal and social functioning not sufficiently addressed. It was in this early post-war period, with its growing focus on constitutional dispositions to depression, that a number of researchers searching for cures for depression focused on some curious biological domains.

Centuries of mistreatment towards depressives was recalled as patients were subjected to some barbaric potential 'cures' such as the removal of gonads, tonsils, uteri (Galen might have approved of this effort), teeth and intestines among other body parts.[53] Some unfortunates were rendered comatose with insulin, put to sleep for days, made hypothermic or were injected with a concoction of different substances. Ewen Cameron, a psychiatrist from Montreal, developed a technique to brainwash patients with the optimistic hope that faulty memory traces could be reprogrammed. Some of his patients underwent repeated ECT to the point of forgetting their names or becoming incontinent but alas with no success, although suspicions about his medical integrity should be considered when we take into account his work being sponsored by those well-known medical philanthropists, the CIA.[53] As many as 50,000 operations were mobilized for the treatment of depression, many of which could barely be justified.

So How Did We Arrive at the Psychiatric Classifications That We Have Today?

Between the years 1917 and 1970, the USA embraced psychotherapy with gusto and the number of psychiatrists in practice grew enormously. A therapeutic culture grew out of the blurring of the boundaries between 'normality' and non-normality and it was not until the 1960s that the practice began to fall out of favour. There were a number of reasons for this reassessment.[55] In the 1950s, the process of scientific falsification was in vogue and the nebulous nature of dynamic psychiatry did not lend itself to the development of objective verification. The movement was simply out of step with these new scientific priorities. During the 1950s, mental patients began to be deinstitutionalized and this meant that a group of patients with more severe disorders were released, often requiring more robust treatment than analysis. In the US alone, the number of institutionalized mental patients dropped by 470,000 between 1955 and 1980. Moreover, the growing protest movement developed a psychiatric arm with much of the previous theory being criticized by prominent psychiatrists like Szasz and Laing, and changing sexual mores meant that the importance of the repression of sexual instinct lost a degree of relevance.

Public embarrassment on social issues such as the disease status of homosexuality emphasized that psychiatric diagnosis was wrapped up in social constructions of deviance. A new model was needed that would medicalize the discipline and legitimize mental health practice and research. As such, specific, discrete and quantifiable diagnostic criteria were formulated. This allowed professionals to aggregate cases, employ the use of statistics and pull their discipline onto an equal footing with other branches of medicine. This new diagnostic culture meant that problems in ordinary life as well as more severe illnesses had to be reconceptualized in diagnostic form so that there was a key for clinicians to refer to. This was supported by a growth in third party insurance payments for psychological trauma where greater accountability and diagnostic certainty were required. You quite simply cannot reimburse continua. Moreover, government programmes that funded an increasing amount of psychotherapy also required categorical accountability. President Carter's 1978 commission on mental health stated that psychiatry was in serious jeopardy, since there was simply inadequate case finding methodology. It was difficult to know who was and who was not depressed or schizophrenic or bipolar?

With regard to the actual process of categorization, there was much rancor and disagreement in the discipline.[56] The problem was that many psychodynamic practitioners felt that careful descriptive diagnosis was at best irrelevant and at worst anathema to good clinical work. There was a concern that such diagnostic criteria might be a greater help to people wishing to commodify mental illness rather than address the needs of the patients themselves.

The process began officially in 1974. Robert Spitzer was appointed by APA President-elect Judd Marmor to be chairman of a task-force on nomenclature and statistics. The previous diagnostic guide required revision and the new guide (DSMIII) was conceptualized as a defense of the medical model. To eliminate the possibility of false positives (diagnosis of an illness to people who did not actually have that illness) and false negatives (no diagnosis of an illness to those who did actually have that illness), it was decided that mental disorders should be narrowly defined. What was publicly visible was given more prominence than what was privately inferred, and hence a direct challenge to the precepts of psychoanalysis. As such, this draft document was attacked on a number of grounds, particularly its lack of clinical relevance and explanatory power, since this new manual did not actually address the factors that caused mental distress. It simply described these different mental disorders. The need to achieve consensus, was for reasons discussed earlier, considered more important than the causes of these various mental illnesses and so the resulting manual came to be symptom-based. Spitzer contested that a diagnostic manual based on 'unproven' causes would splinter the discipline at a time when unity was necessary.

Every time a criticism was launched (and there were many, usually by a district branch of the APA), a task force would make a show of taking account of the criticism without effectively changing their approach. As such, there was widespread umbrage within the discipline against the essentially wholesale removal of psychoanalysis from the psychiatric statute. This new system was refuted by a great number of practitioners from within the discipline, probably a majority, but was pushed through due to the actions of a powerful minority of the APA elite.[55] This new system of criteria may have had dire consequences for psychoanalysis but it allowed new branches of mind sciences like cognitive behavioural therapy, with a focus on discrete symptoms, to flourish. The careful description of symptoms grew to be taken as an adequate psychiatric assessment and formed a narrower perspective that reduced the importance of family dynamics and social factors.

DSM-III has since been translated into more than 20 languages and has grown to become the centerpiece of the knowledge base of American Psychiatry. The DSM description of depression provided in Chapter 1, together with that of dysthymia, bipolar disorder and many others, is the result of these machinations. Through teaching and psychiatric practice over recent years, this system has come to be seen more and more as a natural code; almost as if it was not constructed on non-clinical terms. As Bourdieu[57] noted, every established order tends to produce the naturalization of its own arbitrariness and there are few clearer cases of this than with psychiatric diagnosis. As with other diseases, the symptoms of depression have come to be viewed with greater importance than that which actually causes those symptoms, hence the gradual disintegration of the reactive/endogenous dichotomy that emphasized the causal nature of the illness. The involvement of the pharmaceutical industry has also played a part in the focus on the symptomatology of the depressive diseases. The growth of the antidepressant industry and the growth of the practice of providing antidepressants, regardless of the perceived cause of the illness, have reinforced this practice.

In the US in the 1980s, a very strong lay advocacy group, the National Alliance for the Mentally Ill gained influence in the US congress and the central theme of this organization was that mental illnesses are biological-based brain disorders. The importance of such institutions should not be removed from modern concepts of mental diseases and have helped to shift the psychodynamic influence on faulty parenting practices towards biological factors beyond the control of the sufferer. This has had a major impact regarding issues of responsibility and who we actually 'blame' for depression. It could be construed as beneficial for sufferers, since the way that they are viewed may change; people may be less likely to ascribe depression as a lack of moral strength or laziness or some such designation. However, as will be discussed in later chapters, this is not necessarily beneficial when attempting to understand the political, social and economic factors that can influence the course of depression. A singular focus on the biological can minimize these issues and, in doing so, play a direct role in the continued growth in prevalence over recent years.

What we can see from the concepts of depression through the ages, and especially in recent years, is that there have been a number of different medical definitions and lay beliefs regarding depression. What we can be sure of is that no single one of these representations of depression is 'natural' or objectively defined as we understand the term. Some parties will benefit from defining mental illness in certain terms and it is not always the patients.

Stigma and Depression: A History of Individualism

As touched upon earlier, the strong sociopolitical history of individualism in the US, particularly, has had important implications for the stigma associated with depressive illness. A large Christian evangelical movement swept the country in the first half of the nineteenth century infusing religion with new elements of individualism. Preachers like Henry Ward Beecher spread the message that individuals had to begin to find God within themselves.[58] Protestantism came to be boosted by a new individualist ethos.

With the onset of modernism and with enlightenment thinking placing such an emphasis on scientific rigor and quantifiable measurement, it was a short step to locating that which sciences did not or could not know within the individual. Since we would eventually understand the exterior world, this shifted the responsibility for the unknowable to people rather than the contexts in which people lived.[54] Towards the end of the Victorian era, the idea of personal character, a judgment defined by the adherence to moral or religious guidance, was superseded by the more self-contained concept of the personality. Social and political problems really began to be understood in personal and psychological terms and such movements like mesmerism and positive thinking came to represent popular 'cures' to the ills of the personality. Such a focus on individuality was no doubt influenced by experiences in the new cities that were growing around the country. Where hysteria had established a prominence in European psychiatric thinking, Neurasthenia, through men like George Beard, came to be popular in the US. This represented a form of exhaustion or a paralysis of the will and could be seen to share many of the symptoms in common with what we know now as depression. A therapeutic ethos grew to address these individuals and their individual problems and return them to the workforce, cured.

There were enormous material gains and wealth to be made in the US in the nineteenth century. The idea that great prosperity was open to anyone so long as they had the right work ethic became fundamental to US culture. This is the great self-sustaining myth in the US and is brutally effective since it will always, by definition, have supporters among the powerful elite. However as a result of the political, social and economic restrictions based on class, race, gender and other demographics, the probability of sustained success are very much slanted towards a very particular demographic within this culture. However, this culture of the self has been promulgated by the cultural elite for many years. Phineas Quimby, an important figure in the late Victorian mental health movement, lectured that 'all good things are found within'. Mary Baker Eddy of the New Thought practitioners argued that people could harness the power they had within and use it to take control of the material world. In the world of the mesmerists and the New Thought practitioners, there were no social and political barriers to material success and mental health. Any alienation felt by the monumental move to capitalism and consumerism could be compensated by the knowledge that such riches are open to all.

Particularly in the US, mental ill-health came to be defined as an absence of personal initiative and an inability to work. This was a sickness and this was what mental health practitioners should address. In the early part of the twentieth century, the concepts like 'psyche' and 'mind' were reified by the mental health movement and moved into the colloquial vernacular. By factoring out social and historical influences and medicalizing and individualizing personal problems, the early mental health movement moved concepts of mental health in line with capitalism and the growing importance of consumerism in the West.

Corporatism and psychology grew in parallel in these early years of the twentieth century. It was in the particular interests of corporate and political elites that the importance of the self was promulgated through society. In the US, the disenfranchisement of organized labor was seen as a major necessity in order to achieve sustained corporate success and so individualizing citizens and removing the importance of the social was important not only for the creation of a culture of consumption but also national and international corporate competition. If citizens could be persuaded through advertising, media and legislation that communalism and community were outmoded and indeed dangerous concepts, and that their problems and difficulties were related not to the social or political but to their personal circumstances and their personalities, then they could establish an ethos where consumer rather than political solutions would be the answer.

Consumer choice came to be elevated to the highest of patriotic values, a proxy measure for personal, individual freedom and choice. It became one of the defining aspects of what it meant to be an American. Advertising thrives on individualist and liberationist dogma and during the rise of communism, the action of expressing personal choice through consumption was almost seen as a blow against the enemy.[54] Viewed from this context, depression is an illness that interferes with personal and moral freedom. Unlike many physical illnesses, it is very much an anti-American disease. Individualist ideology states that we are all responsible for the good and bad fortune that we encounter and that dispositional characteristics control this fortune. Simply put, depressives must be at fault somehow for not embracing the American dream, for failing to make the most of their situation and letting themselves fall into this cycle of negativity. As individualism has grown over the last 150 years, so too has the likelihood that depressives would be stigmatized as being responsible for their illness. After all if they decide to mope around rather than be positive then that had to be viewed as their prerogative.

Depression is a disease that can grow within, insidiously, to the point where a sufferer's entire outlook is coloured by the illness. Should one's body be overtaken by a physical illness then this could be excused, since the physical freedom of the sufferer would be compromised but not necessarily the personal and moral sense that they had freedom to live their life as they wish. This is not the case with depression. Personal and moral freedom is usually removed by an illness that often leaves no physical symptoms. Freedom is the last word that most depressives would use to describe their sense of being when they are depressed. This makes the suffering experience a particularly un-American suffering.

Depression also violates the foundational work ethic deeply ingrained in US culture. It violates the belief that hard work and 'pulling your socks up' is simply not enough sometimes. Free market ideology is rife again in the US and the UK and to have faith in the free market and the possibilities afforded everyone under these conditions requires a degree of incomprehension towards those that life has not treated with such beneficence. It is the essence of competition that there will be winners and losers and many of those who arrive on the positive side of that equation are encouraged to rationalize those who have suffered by ascribing attributions of personal responsibility. This belief system contributes to the stigma felt by depressed patients, the archetypes of those rejecting and rejected by the American dream.

What Is Stigma and Why Does It Occur?

So far I have provided a description of some of the principal themes in modern history that have influenced both lay and medical concepts of depression. I have discussed the relationship between growing cultures of individualism and how it relates to the way that depression is represented. In this section, I will outline in more detail how this history might have carried through to substantially affect the current attitudes of people with and without depression. Why is there such heavy stigma associated with depression and what does it mean for our approach to treating the illness?

The issue of stigma is complex and it leads to unjust behaviours and discrimination. It can affect personal identity and social interactions and contributes to social isolation, delays in help seeking and personal distress. It can lead to feelings of guilt, anger and anxiety and is a pervasive phenomenon. Stigma can come from family members, from work colleagues, from health care professionals, educators and members of the general community.[59] It is not unusual for people with mental health disorders to refuse to seek help or to disclose an edited version of their illness and suffering should they feel stigmatized by their disease. Elderly patients with major depression are particularly prone to this discontinuation of treatment via stigma.[60] Stigma can be both felt and enacted, with those feeling stigmatized not necessarily party to actual discrimination from others. The stigma associated with mental health has changed very little in the last 50 years and has contributed negatively and significantly to social exclusion.[61] Indeed it is not uncommon for enacted stigma to lead to the loss of opportunities at work.[62]

Stigma, the Entertainment Media and Mental Illness

Modern media and film has a role to play in our concepts of mental illness generally and a cursory analysis of representations of mental illness does not provide particularly positive findings. Research has shown that when current psychotic symptoms are controlled, there is no difference in recent violent behaviour between patients and never-treated community residents and that only 3% of mentally ill patients are considered dangerous to others. Nevertheless, nearly half of all press coverage of the mentally ill is disproportionately focused on how dangerous such people are. There is an obvious disparity between the actual danger and the danger that one might perceive if exposed to the media.

Many of the misconceptions about mental illness and the treatment of those with mental health problems result from images of mental illness and therapists routinely depicted on film and television.[63] No other art form is so pervasive and we often have little conscious awareness of the huge influence of the entertainment media. This is particularly important when we consider that many people can be uninformed about mental illness. Most of us have probably watched films where a serendipitous bang on the head magically improves a character's personality. Or perhaps the sentimental liberal humanist portrayal of the mentally ill might see them as happy clowns or buffoons where a little bit of freedom from the shackles of the mental health system magically cures them from the evil constraints that were causing their illness.

The general portrayal of mental illness tends to be misleading although that can perhaps be expected, since the function of film is not to educate but to scare, titillate and act as a vehicle for dramatic effect. Wedding and Niemiec[63] isolated core myths regarding mental illness and film. For instance, harmless eccentricity is frequently labelled as mental illness but labelling mental illness as nothing more than harmless eccentricity might well contribute to the idea that this might be the case with many mental disorders. If they are simple eccentricities then surely they cannot be serious disorders that require treatment and sympathy? Such portrayals minimize the suffering of the patient and justifies disparaging attitudes to the serious and prolonged difficulties that many mental health patients experience.

Hollywood films can perpetuate curious beliefs regarding the mental illness spectrum. One such key misunderstanding is the message that 'love can conquer all', a message that is often exhibited in films about mental illness; this idea that with enough loving care and support, people with mental illness can overcome their difficulties and return to society as functioning healthy members. Now while I would agree that having a supportive social network is crucial for many patients with mental illness, 'love' itself is not a panacea for these disorders. To suggest that it is might placate the sentimentalists among us but it manifestly reduces the complexity of the issue and again can contribute to feelings of insufficiency on the part of carers and families. It further influences concepts of mental illness as mild mood fluctuations that can be cured with a bit of tender loving care.

The victims of mental illness are often portrayed as aggressive, unpredictable and dangerous with psychiatrists commonly essayed as inept or manipulative. Horror films are particularly prescient when portraying the psychiatric patient as homicidal and/or fundamentally dangerous and I have lost count of the number of horror films that have used mental illness as a convenient vehicle to explain the most gruesome atrocities. In fact the more able film directors know how to use these concepts of mental illness to pander to the anxieties of their viewers, anxieties that are often driven by disproportionate media representations in the first instance. This is perfectly understandable from the view of generating thrilling entertainment but less so if we are seeking to minimize the misconceptions associated with mental illness.

On occasion, a representation of a mental illness like depression may be reasonably accurate but the need to leave the audience with a smile on their face as they exit the cinema means that pat resolutions and happy endings fail to realize either the true seriousness of the illness or a realistic outcome. Films like *Scent of a Woman* spring to mind in this case. Some films can portray treatment as punishment as was the case with the use of ECT in *One Flew Over the Cuckoos Nest*. This has contributed to the fear and trepidation over what is now one of the safest and most effective treatments for very severe depression.

When we talk about the mental illness myths that are portrayed on film, it is important to reflect on all mental illnesses, be they depression, bipolar disorder, schizophrenia, personality disorders, obsessive compulsive disorder or any other illness. When the public go to the cinema or rent a video, and are exposed to damaging or unhelpful myths regarding a given mental illness, the effect of these myths may be long lasting and influence their beliefs about mental illness in general. Unless they have experience of specific disorders, many people may not know the spectra of specific mental illnesses and nor should they. As such, many of the myths they are exposed to may be applied to the generic category of 'mental disorders' and so concepts relating to a mental health care facility or therapeutic relationship for schizophrenia may be applied to depression.

Many people are not exposed to mental disorders through the everyday course of their lives and films and television may well be their primary source of information. As such, there is an immense responsibility on those who create and screen these images to make them as accurate as possible. Unfortunately this responsibility does not square very well with the financial imperatives of film studios whose sense of responsibility generally stretches to expanding their box office. The real extent of the stigma generated from these representations is difficult to quantify but we would not need Einstein to discern the very real threat of salacious, violent and despicable acts being repeatedly explained by inaccurate representations of mental disorders. When we understand the increasing amount of time that people (particularly children) watch television and films, it is perhaps not difficult to understand why there has been little decrease in the stigma associated with mental illnesses in the last 50 years.

Stigma and Depression

As the brief history of depression showed at the beginning of the chapter, the medical and religious firmament should not be patting itself on the back with regards to how it has represented and treated depressives through the years. Two thousand years of humiliation, mistrust, outcasting, punishment and general antipathy will leave its effect on how we currently feel about people with depression. Concepts are passed on from generation to generation and the ideas of depressives having 'sinned against God' or having a sexual aetiology to their illness does not necessarily encourage people with the disorder to proudly put their hands up and identify themselves with a history of supposed malingerers, sinners, sexual miscreants, and lazy and self-obsessed serial complainers, who drain the personal and financial resources of others.

Common reactions to depression (or variants on these themes) are considered below and hearing these from people with little experience of the illness is not unusual. Indeed, sometimes these are said with sanctimonious and pious glee. Many of the prompts are used by family/friends/employers to try to shake the sufferer out of their depressive stupor but are usually about as effective as telling a heart attack or stroke victim to 'run it off'. The real reason many of these comments are so incredibly unhelpful is that they presuppose that depression is a choice of the sufferer and that they can choose not to be depressed should they so wish.

"What have you got to feel so miserable about, you have a roof over your head and a good job?"

This comment supposes that depression itself must automatically be related in some way to the worldly possessions of the sufferer, and that there could be no reason that the sufferer would be depressed other than what they possess financially.

Many episodes of depression are related to life events or are exacerbated by life events in some way but some are not. For both kinds of depression, having a given set of possessions or lifestyle is usually not enough to protect the sufferer from slipping towards the illness. We can be sure that once the sufferer has tipped over into the clinical syndrome of major depression, it is utterly irrelevant to link their suffering and pain to a roof and a safe job. In the abstract sense, it makes about as much sense as saying to someone 'what have you got to have a heart attack about, you have a nice job and house'. Heart disease and depression are illnesses, not life choices.

"Look at all the starving children in the world, don't you know how lucky you are?"

As anyone who has suffered major depression will know, it is usually a horrendous and debilitating illness that infuses every aspect of the sufferer's life. The last thing you feel is lucky, regardless of how many objective reasons there are for people to consider you lucky. Comments like those above lead to further guilt and self recrimination, two unpleasant properties that depressives are usually not short of in the first instance. Depressed people usually know that being a starving child is unpleasant but there is no linear relationship to the number of bad things happening to you and how bad you feel. Depression is an illness and it is very different for different people in different places. There is no rule of thumb that stipulates that x amount of bad things will lead to y amount of feeling bad. Exhorting a diabetic patient with such a prompt would probably just lead to confusion on the part of the patient but such a reaction will not be experienced by the depressive patient because they often share the same beliefs systems as those doing the exhorting. As such, it can simply lead to further guilt and worthlessness.

"I know many people worse off than you."

Ditto. See above. 'Worse off' is a subjective term and the comparison is futile. At the root of this is the basic belief that the person saying it does not understand depression itself to be a worthy item to add to a prospective list of good and bad things that are happening to you. This exhortation relies on good old fashioned logic. Being 'worse off' is an irrelevance, since many depressives no longer have the capacity to 'objectively' judge whether things are that bad or not. Appeals to this kind of logic are futile and will more likely intensify the distress experienced by the depressive. Logic needs to be removed from any appeal because depression is not a logical state, it is an illness that removes the capacity to balance the normal pros and cons of life.

The above perception boils down to the fact that this person, and many others, simply have no idea of the agony, pain, hopelessness and despair that often characterizes depression. If they did then they would probably be prompted to think 'actually there are very few people worse off than you at this present time'. I think that a great many people suffering a severe depressive episode would give away all of their worldly possessions for the guarantee of feeling human again, to leave the 'black hole' behind.

"Don't worry, it will all come out in the wash."

This is a worthwhile statement for someone who is feeling a little down because their pet is ill or because they have been admonished by their boss. Illnesses tend not to come out in the wash. Most often people with serious major depression will require some kind of treatment in order for them to go into remission and, at the very least, this will hasten the process. While it is perfectly reasonable to assume that some people may eventually recover without medical help, this is not a serious option and should not be recommended. People with depression should seek medical help from their general practitioner because otherwise they could endure a prolonged period of despair. There is a feeling among some members of the public that depression somehow fails to warrant treatment. This is because it is a 'mental' illness rather than a physical illness and so is simply a reflection of dispositional weakness of character. Depression is actually a physical and a mental illness and it needs to be addressed as soon as possible to minimize the possibility of more recurrent and severe episodes in the future. The message is, seek help.

Pull your socks up.

Ah yes, now we are getting to the bare bones of the problem. I suspect that some depressives would be quite wealthy were they to be given a pound for every time they heard this. Regarding treatment for depression, the views of the public are interesting. 36% of people interviewed believed that you 'have to pull yourself together' if you are depressed.[64] This fundamentally betrays the belief that the sufferer has a choice to be depressed or not. Depression is characterized here as some form of extended self pity, wallowing in a misery that they could easily choose to leave behind. This is one of the most frustrating things that the sufferer can hear because (a) it shows a fundamental misunderstanding of the severity of their suffering, (b) it suggests that they could stop this suffering should they choose to and (c) that they do not want to recover and are happy with their life as it currently is.

Anyone who knows the pain of depression knows that this is an insult. However, many depressed people can become so dependent on the people around them that they are in a position where they have to absorb and accept such comments. Very many are unlikely to have the energy or the inclination to argue the point.

People obviously want their loved ones to be well and it is often easier to blame the sufferer for their behaviour than to accept and process the knowledge that they, as the loved one, are completely powerless to address the despair of this person who is probably changing beyond recognition. Comments like this are more likely to prompt people to suffer in silence than to make them consult a GP. After all, if my husband or daughter or best friend does not believe me, why should a general practitioner?

There is a theme behind the above comments and that is the simple failure to acknowledge that depression is an illness. Until this is appreciated then patients and their loved ones are going to continue to struggle. Exhortations and appeals are quite simply not enough to bring people out of major depressions because they are based on fundamental inaccuracies.

There are a number of fundamental myths that pervade the experience of depression in the west and they are directly responsible for the reactions above as well as the stigma, shame and anxiety that haunt the experience of depression.

We All Get Down Sometimes

This is true but we do not all get depressed sometimes. Depression is not a transitory state of mild dissatisfaction in relation to minor difficulties. The creation of some imaginary scale with clinical depression at one end and slightly perturbed at the other is unhelpful and inaccurate, despite the contentions of recent professionals.[65] Depression does not exist on a spectrum that incorporates natural reactions to everyday difficulties because, for one, the symptoms are often different. In the vast majority of cases, transient sadness and feeling 'down in the dumps' is exactly that. People will feel sad or they will be upset or they will feel slightly low in mood. They will not, however, usually feel apathy, anhedonia, fatigue and emptiness. They will not experience a feeling of lingering despair or dread and it is unlikely that they will experience serious fluctuations in their weight and sleeping patterns. People can suffer clinical depression without feeling apathy and emptiness but they are very common symptoms of the depressive illness and they are simply not experienced during transitory sadness. Indeed, by definition, transitory sadness shows an ability to feel affect, to care and to hurt. These functions are often not available to the depressive and it is a qualitatively different experience. About 67% of people believe that the support system of family and friends should be the source of help for people with depression.[66] Only a few people recommended seeing a psychiatrist for major depression. This support system can be extremely helpful and in many cases utterly essential in the recovery from depression. However again this result betrays an understanding of depression as a mood rather than an illness. I doubt such surveys for cancer or heart disease would recommend the family as the source of help for patients and while this parallel may appear extreme, I believe it is fundamentally fair. A refusal to accept depression as an illness will continue to contribute to the often monumental distress and poor recovery of depressives.

It is true that the clinical definition of major depression is an arbitrary abstraction. However, that does not preclude the existence of a distinct illness entity. The bottom line is that there is debate within the mental health sciences regarding the nature and form of depression or depressions and we are nowhere near the point of fully comprehending the biological, psychosocial or nosological issues involved. It may well be that a dimensional model of the illness is more appropriate than a categorical model but starting the scale at transiently feeling down in the dumps for a few hours or an evening could be a dangerous avenue to travel down. Such conceptualizations play a role in the generation of ignorance and stigma that surrounds the illness and could contribute to reduced help-seeking. No matter how you choose to cut the categorical cake, it still exists and the arbitrary definition does not denude this.

This failure to separate the illness from the vernacular appropriation of depression can be traced back to the birth of the mental health sciences. As mentioned, the psychoanalytic movement helped to cement the relationship between neurotic and normal behaviour so that both were variants of common developmental processes. This had the benefit of making people appreciate that anyone could become mentally ill if they were exposed to the right stimuli and that people with mental disorders were not necessarily a breed apart from normal people. On the whole this was a positive. However in the case of common mental disorders like depression, it is also likely to have played a role in cementing the idea that general dissatisfaction with lifestyles is a milder form of depression as they both now received the same treatment. This dissatisfaction with the vicissitudes of life was given clinical credibility and with it, the barriers between everyday up and downs and major depression, were eroded. A simple failure to separate these two distinct experiences has contributed to a lack of sympathy towards sufferers of depression over the years.

There is a need to educate the public about this particular aspect of depression in order to address this stigma associated with the 'we all get sad, what is special about you' doctrine. Yes, negative events can lead to crises and act as precipitating factors in the development of depression. Difficult circumstances like financial strain, abuse, gender issues and occupational stresses, among others, all relate to depression and can play a fundamental role. However, they are not necessary and depression can, for some people, develop in what seems like a vacuum. Depression can just happen. Sometimes, from nowhere, and with no warning or rational justification, the most savage and brutal despair will descend upon a sufferer and this aspect of the illness needs to be more fully appreciated in order to generate greater public empathy. Sometimes, it simply does not matter what you have done and how you have done it, many people will become terribly depressed despite living in a virtual paradise.

This seeming randomness can be very difficult to understand. It can also be a little frightening and this fear can make it easier to blame the sufferer rather than understand that a harrowing illness can strike from nowhere. Enacted stigma can emanate from the characteristics of those who stigmatize as much as representations of the stigmatized. John Updike, in reference to people who were stigmatized as a result of a disfiguring skin disease, believed that people turning away from those with such skin diseases stemmed from a fleeting identification with the person who is afflicted. The afflicted individual represents our own vulnerability and imperfection and our real lack of autonomy and control over many of the forces that shape our lives. This desire to link depression with life events in a logical, systematic way may be influenced by just such attitudes, making those of us lucky enough not to be affected by the illness keen to link the illness to dispositional characteristics. When you experience mental illness, a new vulnerability opens up that stays with you. It sometimes destroys previous concepts of cause and effect, of illness and aetiology.

Strength and Depression

There is a popular sense that if you are a strong person then depression simply cannot happen to you. For many, strong people do not get depressed because they can bear the vicissitudes of life, they cope with whatever life throws at them and they do it because they have an implicit strength. However, depression is not related to how strong you are and some of the most powerful people in history, people like Winston Churchill, have suffered from crippling bouts of depression.

Many people with depression are not fond of the concept that they have capitulated under conditions that another may endure and sufferers will often keep quiet for as long as possible. Having talked to depressed patients, much of the stigma is acutely felt by those who perceive themselves to be weak. Again we can reduce this attitude down to the basic belief or lack of belief in the status of depression as an illness. If you fail to accept it as an illness then it is usually contextualized as a character trait. However recent figures have suggested that as many as 50%[22] of people will suffer from depression at some point in their life. Whether all of these people develop severe depression is debatable but if we follow the logic that depression only affects the weak then that is a lot of weak people.

Biology, Stigma and Depression

As mentioned, many people with depression are not fond of the idea that they have failed to withstand challenges that another person may cope with and so there is a self-preservative interest in implicating chemical processes beyond our control. This is especially the case in Western societies where the ethos of personal responsibility and the 'just world hypothesis' are subscribed to by so many. During the 1980s, a strong US lay advocacy group, the National Alliance for the Mentally Ill (NAMI), gained influence in the US congress and the central theme of the organization was that mental illnesses were brain-based disorders that resulted from biological factors. This biological focus meant that responsibility for their suffering could be removed from the patient. Factors beyond the role of the sufferer were implicated and this has proved to be a useful way of reducing the stigma associated with the illness, especially in Western culture. Of course there are very important biological findings that relate to the illness, not least with respect to genetics, cerebral blood flow and antidepressant action, and the NAMI are right to emphasise these.

While the NAMI use strictly medical and biological terminology in their information pamphlets, research has suggested that the public still prefer social explanations for the causes of depression and fail to reflect the legitimizing practice of biological explanations.[67] Recent research with college students suggests that people recognized biological, psychological and environmental explanations of depression. Endorsement of the biological model tended to be empowering and predicted greater help-seeking behaviour and had a positive impact on stigma.[67] Adopting the psychological model increased the blame towards participants who had depression and this suggests support for anti-stigma organizations like the NAMI.

Implicating the biological basis of depression is effective with regard to reducing the stigma of personal weakness. However, despite there being strong evidence implicating biological processes in depressions, an excessive emphasis on this will denigrate the role of social, psychological and political organizational factors and this can be a profoundly deleterious consequence. The ways in which this can work to disable sufferers are discussed further in Chapter 5.

Different people hold different beliefs based on their personal experiences with the illness. Some sufferers may prefer to attribute their depression to psychological causes for the very reason that this means they do have some aspect of responsibility or control over it. The attributions that are formed depends on a number of factors including the need for control, the need not to be blamed for the condition and the desire to avoid stigmatization and the latter need is one that can be partly ameliorated by moving responsibility to biological factors.

What Does the Public Think About Depression Today?

Work has been carried out to try to ascertain exactly what people generally know about depression. It is interesting that only 39% of the public recognized vignettes of depressed people as actually being depressed and that 11% thought that the cases had a physical disorder.[24] Other work suggests that a US sample of the general public were reasonably knowledgeable about mood symptoms but less so regarding the somatic changes that often represent the symptoms of depression.

On the topic of stigma, 35% of the general population would not rent a room to someone with depression and 42% would refuse to recommend them for a job, probably in fear that the participant would not be able to keep the job or manage the tasks that the role would entail.[68] One of the more interesting aspects of this research with a German sample was that there appeared to be no changes over the last decade with regard to people's attitudes to those with depression. It was suggested that a tendency to act with irritation and anger towards depressives had actually increased slightly and so this suggests that public initiatives to address the stigma surrounding the illness are a long way from being effective, certainly in Germany at least. The participants reported that the desire to distance themselves from someone with depression was as strong in 2001 as it was in 1991 and this inertia showed no particular variance with regard to such socioeconomic factors as gender, age or education. This kind of research that looks at public attitudes to depression over time is useful as it allows us to understand and address the effectiveness of initiatives designed to make the public more understanding and sympathetic to those suffering with illnesses like depression.

Regarding the causes of depression, recent work has shown that 48% of people believe that depression is a reaction to an external problem[64] and that it is due more to psychosocial circumstances than biological causes.[69] While this can often be the case, such strong beliefs in causality may not leave room for the high number of depressed people whose depression has not come as a response to external events, the so-called endogenous depressives. Such a belief may be unlikely to predispose many of this 48% to a sympathetic attitude when faced with someone with whom they could see no reason as to why they should be depressed. Many depressed people cannot find such a reason and feel doubly stigmatized, first of all for having the illness, and second, for their failure to isolate 'valid' reasons for their depression. Work has also confirmed that depression is perceived by many to be a normal extension of the feelings that most people experience. This confirms the earlier discussion of the link between minor ailments and clinical depression.[66]

Regarding treatment, other work has shown that for people suffering with depression, psychiatrists and psychologists are rated less highly than general practitioners,[24] although in the UK the majority of the public would feel embarrassed about visiting their GP for depression. The public have had a tendency to perceive psychiatric medicine as more harmful than helpful[70] and a skeptical attitude towards mental health practitioners is age-old. As far back as Greek antiquity, sophists, party to behavioural and lingual knowledge not immediately available to the lay person, were often seen as manipulating essential public health institutions such as the practices of law and health. A part of the stigma associated with being a service user of a mental health system, whether it is a general practice, psychiatrist or psychologist, is that you are now part of this context that uses rhetorical services and specialized, secret and manipulative knowledge. People under this care can be seen as being agents of mental health practitioners and can become objects of skepticism and mistrust by association. They have crossed over to the metaphorical 'other side' and have removed themselves from the unwritten contract of living their lives within the straightforward terms of the everyman. For some, this can also play a role in concepts of stigma and a desire not to receive treatment and medical recognition for a mental health problem.

How Do Depressed People Experience Stigma?

Stigma dominates the experience of depression and upward of 70% of people with depression do not seek care. There are effective treatments available but most people will avoid visiting a health professional regarding their depression and this strong sense of perceived stigma is a powerful barrier to help-seeking behaviour. Taking antidepressant medication can confirm the subjective feeling that they are failures who are unable to cope with the problems that everyone else seems to be able to manage. Taking antidepressants for a prolonged period often makes sufferers feel pathetic; reinforcing negative views that they may have of themselves. Many people forget that it is not only non-depressed people that hold negative attitudes to the depressed but people who become depressed themselves. Indeed, compared to those who seek treatment, those who fail to seek treatment for their illness are more likely to be embarrassed if friends or relatives find out about their depression and treatment.[71] Moreover, feelings of stigma have been shown to be significantly associated with the severity of depression.

A number of focus groups and interviews showed that those who suffered with depression and anxiety had a strong sense that people were not sensitive to their problems.[26] When we consider the earlier figures on public beliefs regarding the causes and remedies for depression and the strong history of stigmatization associated with the disease, then this is perhaps understandable. People with depression are stigmatized and in many instances people are not sympathetic to their problems. It should be emphasized that these feelings are not necessarily a further symptom of the illness or a cognitive distortion or error on the part of the sufferer. Because of a history of stigmatization, ignorance and misunderstanding concerning the disease and its causes, sympathy for depressives is often in short supply. Many of these patients feel a pervasive sense of being different, of being misunderstood and of feeling isolated, and feel that their general practitioners are too busy to address such a trivial illness as depression. This may or may not be the case but there can be little doubt that many people feel that their time in health consultation at their local practice is severely limited.

Common feelings of low self-worth often mean that depressed people do not feel worthy of their doctor's time and this, combined, with perceptions of doctor's attitudes and the limited time available in consultation contributes to a real lack of recognition and treatment of depression. Opening up to a general practitioner, especially a GP that you may not know, is not easy for many people and so the next best option is not to provide any information or limited information in the hope that a doctor can diagnose them without trudging through the difficult and shameful feelings. Other concerns might be about having the stigma of an emotional problem 'on record' and how this might impact upon such future lifestyle issues like parental fitness, custody and occupational suitability. Indeed the example of a severely depressed woman who was told by a social worker that, as a result of her 'resorting' to prescription drugs, she was vulnerable to having her child taken from her if the child experienced problems, highlights a not uncommon source of concern.[72] Many patients simply want someone to acknowledge that they are struggling and this should be the least a patient can expect from a visit to a health professional.

Of course stigma is not the only reason that people keep their depression to themselves and fail to tell their general practitioner or family members. Some people are simply unaware that they are suffering from depression and it has been suggested that up to 50% of the untreated depressed did not perceive themselves to have a mental health problem.[71] Then again, many people do not consider depression or the subjective symptoms of depression to constitute a mental health problem with such symptoms as poor sleep patterns, lack of energy and low mood being perceived outside of the domain of mental health.

Concluding Remarks

The Royal College of Psychiatrists in the UK has launched a five-year campaign to reduce stigmatization for people with mental health problems and it has centered around such concepts as open communication, community awareness, education and protection against discrimination. This Defeat Depression Campaign has registered a small but positive change in certain attitudes such as the effectiveness of antidepressants. However, the need for such initiatives continues, especially within a primary care context.

The stigma felt by many with depression is understandable because the consequences of their illness are often minimized or personal blame attached to their actions and behaviour. The public should continue to be informed, perhaps through adverts and programmes in the media and in health care environments, that depression is an illness and that the support system of family and friends, whilst absolutely crucial, is often not enough. Medical treatment is appropriate and necessary in many cases. If a person has little knowledge of depression then they may feel that natural remedies or lifestyle change are the only cures. Taking medication for a prolonged period can make people feel pathetic and weak but such perceptions need to be challenged. A focus on depression as an illness will help us to achieve this. A reformulation of drug use in the context of other chronic conditions like epilepsy and diabetes could help many people to appreciate that it is in the best interests of some patients to undertake lengthy and perhaps even permanent medication for their illness.

Not all antidepressant medications work for everyone and psychological therapies have been shown to benefit many sufferers. Finding the right treatment for the individual is important but breaking down the stigma associated with these treatments is fundamental to any approach to instituting and prolonging recovery. Following agreement to take antidepressant medication, there are a number of factors that can act as barriers to adherence to this treatment and these include the nature of the disease itself; the associated problems with memory, hopelessness and concentration. The stigma related to concepts of the depressed individual as morally weak or flawed, or a general unawareness of the importance of consistently taking the medication could also contribute and should be addressed in any future initiatives to destigmatize the condition.

In recent years, a group of self-help books on depression have emerged. Some of these texts are more helpful than others but the great majority fall foul of the major financial conflict involved in successfully marketing any book on a medical illness. That is, the promise that the book in question will somehow bring about improvement in the sufferers' condition or effect a cure based on a given set of principles contained within the book. The certitude of the language contained in many of these self-help books can support feelings of failure in participants who are unable to achieve the promised or implied successes that should automatically result from following the tenets. Such promises as 'restoration is available to anyone who embarks upon tackling depression thought the suggestions in this book'[72] do not leave much sympathy for those who do not find restitution after following the miracle suggestions. Does this mean the illness is their fault? Do they not want to get better? Do they actually have depression in the first place? When the text in question contains a foreword by the head of SANE, the prominent UK mental health charity, there seems to be little room to disagree with the validity of its conclusions and recommendations. This is one example but there are many others on the market and their promises of immediate restitution should be taken with a king-sized spoonful of salt. Depression can be a particularly idiosyncratic illness experience with different people experiencing different symptoms at different times and with varying magnitude. Since the waiting list for counseling can be long and since there can be such mistrust of antidepressant medications, many resort to these texts that may end up exacerbating the distress associated with the illness.

One other problem that afflicts the community of people suffering from depression, and the way that they are represented, is the disenfranchisement that comes from being afflicted by a disease that can make sufferers so hopeless and helpless. The depressed have little political say due to the restrictions of their disease. You cannot vote if you are not able to leave your house and you will not vote if you do not care whether you wake up or not. This basic principle means that generating a political lobbying effort for depression is more difficult than it is for other illnesses, since many who are suffering the most severe ravages of the condition are unable to contribute to a source of political momentum.

Generally speaking, a focus on depression has always tended to be a focus on the well-being of individual people suffering from depression from a psychological and/or biological perspective. This approach towards depression has the individual as the level of analysis for research and treatment. However, people with depression and their families and friends exist in a society and I have already discussed how important this society can be with regard to the stigma surrounding the illness. The relationships between the political, economic and structural events in society that play a role in the epidemiology of the illness are rarely discussed. However, the well-being and mental and physical health of those who live in society are intimately related to the political, social and economic events that influence what it means to exist within that society. Such a macroscopic perspective tends to be less prominent than the microscopic perspective that focuses on the biology and psychology of the problems that people struggle to cope with in their everyday lives.

Exactly how does modern living in the west relate to the psychological problems and biological predispositions that people exhibit? Before addressing this question in Chapter 5, the next two chapters focus on some of the prominent political, economic and social changes in the post-war era. In the recent era of globalization, such structural changes have had profound consequences for people who struggle with depression on a day to day basis.

II: Globalization

Chapter 3
The New Right and the 1980s

Any discussion of the political changes in the west in recent years can only be truly understood when located in a historical context. Social, political and financial trends have led to what we today refer to as globalization; the ethos around which the central tenets (often unknown or nebulously stated) of international trade, finance, market economics, welfare, social policy and socioeconomic organization are currently organized. Perhaps unusually for a discussion on globalization, I am not going to provide a conceptual definition until the next chapter. The reason is that to understand the evolution of today's international economic and political systems, we need to travel back through recent history, at least as far as the industrial revolution and Victoria's England. Such a history is bound to be brief, excessively so, and so I apologize to historians who note the complexity of their field of study reduced to a rangy skeleton. However, the purpose of such a discussion is to frame current developments and for this purpose it will suffice.

Victoria's England: The Development of Industry and International Trade

In the seventeenth and eighteenth centuries, there was a steady increase in European commerce. The seasonal fairs of medieval Europe were gradually replaced by permanent centers of exchange, the use of bills of exchange and credit. In Amsterdam and London particularly, a culture of moneylenders and commodity dealers and a growth in financial houses became prominent. Gradually a system of national and international credit came to underpin the modern economy. The financial stability and reliability of clients superseded their religious status as the criteria for mercantile relationships and, following the erosion of tariff barriers in the mid-nineteenth century, a new international order of trade arose.

Laissez-faire capitalism took off with a vengeance and the UK government's non-intervention in the Irish famine, with its subsequently tragic consequences, was possibly the most extreme example of this political ethos. The government of the time viewed the Irish famine as the responsibility of the landowners who, generally speaking, did very little to alleviate the massive suffering and fatalities that ensued.

To move the workers from the fields into the factories, a general social and moral consensus had to be created such that rebellion against this development became a moral issue.[73] The 'work ethic' was manufactured to provide the impetus to move workers from the farms to the factories. This ethic served the interests of politicians and preachers in their battle to overcome the primary obstacle that was holding back the development of the world that they wanted to build. They needed to separate the productive effort of UK workers from concepts of personal and family need such that people would work above and beyond what was considered necessary for subsistence. A new approach defined by 'what could be done' rather than 'what was needed' was instituted and the creation of the work ethic framed this process.

The key battle was to prevail over the natural reluctance of would-be factory workers to the discomfort and difficulties of a work regime that they neither needed nor wanted. The work ethic allowed the moral superiority of any kind of lifestyle that supported the wages of labor and this concept was particularly effective at linking human value and occupational status. It should be noted, however, that the work ethic is a particularly European invention. Many historians will concur that such a strategy did not need to be invented in the US since the inherent spirit of enterprise and desire for upward mobility tended to drive the wheels of US industry.

What were previously open fields on which peasants could toil were claimed in ownership by wealthy lords for the development of commercial schemes. By 1873, this process had led to more than 80% of all of the land in the UK coming under the ownership of less than 7000 men. Peasants lost control of what had previously been common land and with it, an independent subsistence. In what was an incredibly swift change in the working culture, the lucky ones were driven into local city factories while others found themselves in the dreaded workhouses. Indeed, modernization itself could be defined by this movement of workers.

The industrial proletariat of the time paid an awful toll as this new class labored in mines and lived in unhealthy, filthy and hastily constructed cities. The 1834 Poor Law Amendment Act sanctioned and, indeed encouraged, the building of workhouses, the last resort for the chronically indigent, where families were separated and adults and children put to work for long and painful working days. These workhouses separated the idle from the workers such that their laziness would not infest the hard-working. In the US, the 'social revolution' drove organized labor in the much same way as it was driven in the UK but without the meager protection offered to the working classes in the UK since in England the Aristocratic tendency was to express a general inertia towards the cut and thrust of market capitalism.

The anti-corn law league was organized around the precept that free trade should have a positive social effect (or at least that is what they maintained publicly) in 'drawing men together, removing the antagonism of race, creed and language, (and) unite us in the bonds of eternal peace'.[74] Together with the movement towards free trade, the birth of consumer society is considered to have occurred in this era with a conspicuous growth in high fashion and the development of shopping and commercial life.

Although these times were characteristically difficult for the working people of Britain, small increments in political capital would point to a better existence in the future. For instance the 1867 Representation of the People Act enfranchised an extra one million urban working class household males.

1900–1945: A Gradual Turn to Social Democracy

The turn of the century brought with it a number of political developments that were designed to improve the often wretched quality of life of much of the UK populous. For instance in 1901, the minimum working age was raised to 12, following continual increments throughout the nineteenth century. The formation of the Labour Party from the Labour Representation Committee in 1906 heralded a third political force in mainstream British Politics and was a party developed as a source of representation for working men. However, it was the Liberal Party that spearheaded developments in quality of life and welfare during this era. The principal of the minimum wage was established in 1909 and the 'people's budget' paid for pension and national insurance with regard to unemployment benefit and health. This was to be jointly paid for by the state, employers and employees. Progressive redistributive taxation was introduced, leading to revolt in the Lords, so much so that the Parliament Act was developed to minimize the power and influence of the second house. Relying on income tax for revenue allowed the abolition of Victorian import duties with the wealthier classes made to bear the brunt of these developments.

The quality of life of UK citizens was improving, although some 30% of people still existed in some degree of poverty in the early twentieth century, with 10% in acute need. Although nostalgic reminiscence suggests otherwise, most people still had a hard life prior to the First World War.

Trade continued to grow and the volume of UK trade was six times greater in 1910 than it had been in Victorian times. The UK and US were particularly protective of their own markets and, as a result, a sevenfold increase in US exports was noted between 1860 and 1914, with imports increasing only fivefold. Trade protectionism was one of the political issues of the day and a source of division within the principal political parties.

Between the wars there was fierce competition in raw material for manufacturing and farm produce and increased national resentments were noted by many politicians, with a concomitant lurch to the right. Assertive national policies were backed, if necessary, by military action, and were the popular consensus of the time and the problems produced by the territorial settlements of the First World War led to large groups of ethnic minorities living on the 'wrong' sides of these recently created national borders.

However, social policy was progressive on both sides of the Atlantic. In the UK, the Unemployment Insurance Act of 1920 included a further 12 million workers. Winston Churchill wanted to link the self-interest of millions of people around the country to the capitalist movement and this was the basis of the 1925 Widows and Old Age Pension's Act. Although industrial disputes were rife in the twenties, with 1926 the worst year for industrial disputes in Britain, unemployment insurance continued to grow, with the 1930 Act removing previous restrictions on claiming benefits. In 1937, the Factories Act continued this upward trend as the hours of work of young persons under the age of 16 were limited to 44 per week. Poverty was still rife but had been abnegated during Baldwin's administration (much like Thatcher's in the 1980s) by counting on the haves in the South East of the country outnumbering the have-nots elsewhere.

In the US, old age and unemployment insurance programmes were not enacted until the 1930s as Roosevelt's New Deal sought to address the devastation wrought by the depression. On the eve of the Second World War, the US pledged more of its national product to social security than any major industrial nation but Roosevelt lost interest in social policy with the onset of the war.

1945–1975: The Post-War Experiment in Social Democracy

While Orwell still had cause to note that England was the most class ridden nation under the sun, social policy appeared to be moving in a more inclusive, egalitarian direction. Following the war, the 1945 Family Allowances Act heralded a direct attack on poverty and meant that an allowance for second and subsequent children would be paid to mothers.

The end of the Second World War saw a Labour administration take office under Clement Attlee and they took a number of enterprises into common national ownership. In 1946, a contributory state retirement pension was paid to all, even those too young to contribute. The UK (like many countries around the world) was fundamentally dependent on the US and 'Marshall Aid' provided the financial impetus for the British Welfare state. The World Bank wrote $2.7 billion of war debts off and the US guaranteed a further $1.3 billion for the French trade deficit, although such benevolence did not spread to countries such as Poland, Hungary and Czechoslovakia, which were to fall under the rule of the USSR.[75] In Japan the reconstruction was informed by New Deal theories of the 1930s and General Macarthur and his aides imposed a liberal constitution and a virtual social revolution. Unfortunately, such munificence was not shown by the US government to its own people. The New Deal had been rejected and/or watered down to the extent that the only post-war national spending commitments were for old age or survivors allowance for soldiers.

Numerous theories expound as to why welfare, in the form of Beveridge's call for the creation of the National Health Service and a commitment to full employment, was heeded after the war and why it was embraced in Europe but so soundly rejected in the US. Some suggested that a welfare state was the means by which the health and morale of a nation could remain bolstered and ready for future conflict, although one might doubt that, after 6 years of war, many people were thinking about preparations for another one. More likely, people can tolerate high taxes following war because they are simply used to it and so social spending is fundamentally more acceptable. However, some analysts believe that, for the US, the war did not actually end as such.[76] The cold war with the USSR meant that this displacement effect did not happen in the US.

Some have suggested that social spending arrives on the back of increases in morality and national unity following prolonged war. Perhaps the UK was more affected in this way as a result of the continual bombing campaigns that its citizens were subjected to. With the exception of such outposts as Pearl Harbour, US citizens on the mainland did not experience this. There was another reason for this difference between the US and the UK. The New Deal failed because, in a fundamental sense, the US was not a democracy. The lack of democratic parties in the South made it difficult to create a regime based on reform. US political institutions made it difficult for innovations in social provision as the US was more infested with patronage-oriented political parties and US political institutions were more fragmented. The profound influence of veteran's associations over matters such as health, insurance and disability programmes worked against the institution of national programmes for non-veterans. Indeed, it was not until the 1960s that the US could boast broad, government-funded health insurance programmes. Further, wartime coalition in the US did not achieve the same degree of control over the economy in the US as the UK coalition did. In the US, the key leadership roles went to military officials and leaders in the business community rather than civil administrators and labor leaders. Indeed, following the war, Senator Joe McCarthy manufactured a powerful campaign based on fear and jingoism, the purpose of which was to undermine these labor leaders, labor rights generally and hence functioning democracy. Aided by such institutions as the FBI and the American Protective League, a conservative business organization, information was provided on labor union activists under the guise of their being 'agents or persons unfriendly to the government'.[77] This was a theme that continued for much of the post-war period with the FBI instituting initiatives to confuse and disrupt the activities of civil liberty and left wing groups.

The UK coalition introduced the conservatives to reforming influences, whereas the 1948 US democratic victory was relatively insignificant because there was no congressional strength for social reform. In the battle against the regulation of working hours, war heroes were paraded across the country speaking against work time reductions. The anticommunist hysteria led to attacks on unionized labor and virulent anti-union legislation was enacted. The fact that in 1930, the Kellogg Company found that a switch to a 6 hour day (to cope with the effects of the depression) led to more productive workers was ignored. The strong individualistic history of the US, already discussed in the previous chapter, also meant that anti-union legislation and minimal social reform were always going to be easier to achieve there than elsewhere.

In post-war Europe, the virulent free market capitalism of the Victorian era was on the defensive and some authors even thought that it had had its time; that it was, as a political and economic system, redundant. The popular post-war belief was that capitalism would give way to socialism. In reality, capitalism was tamed because the governments of the West realized that they needed the support of their own working classes in order to contest and reject the Soviet model of economic organization.[78]

By 1951, the UK government increased housing subsidies and pledged to build an extra 300,000 houses per year. Although education was still class-bound, social reform appeared to be moving in a more inclusive direction. In 1959, Gaitskill, much like Tony Blair 35 years later, tried to radically amend Clause IV but unlike Tony Blair, he failed because the Unions would not allow it. By the late 1950s, the quality of life of UK citizens had improved enough to allow Harold MacMillan to extol his electorate that 'they had never had it so good'. However in the US, a note of warning was sounded in 1961 by Eisenhower who, in his farewell address, noted that democracy had to be guarded against the acquisition of unwarranted influence by the military–industrial complex.

The growing importance of television emphasized the importance of the private household and in the UK in 1963, the abolition of schedule A in tax returns gave a tax subsidy to owner-occupiers, thus rewarding private ownership. While this select group was growing from a low of 10% before the First World War, it would not be until the 1980s that the explosion of home owners would truly be realized. Still, social reform continued to emphasize the quality of life of the majority of UK citizens and in 1965 the Redundancy Payments Act provided redundancy relative to the length of service within a given occupation.

Harold Wilson had ascended the political throne and his middle management style of premiership and a perceived need to create New Britain set the template for the New Labour revolution in the 1990s. In the early 1960s, 70% of the UK public thought that unions were a good thing but this number had dropped to 57% by 1969 and strike ballots and cooling off periods were suggested by the Wilson administration as a way to outflank the conservatives.[75]

In the US, the new post-war spirit of confidence, personal entitlement and acquisitiveness marked the explosion of consumer culture. It was illustrated by a 114% increase in GNP between 1940 and 1960 and the GNP would rocket from $500 billion in 1960 to $1 trillion in 1971. During this time, the US battle against communism on all fronts had led to their becoming embroiled in a messy and awkward war in Vietnam, a war that only stopped when it began to seriously damage their internal economy. Military spending was fuelled by perceptions of the Soviet Nuclear threat and exacerbated by Vietnam. The policy of increased military spending, however, was beneficial on two counts. First, it addressed the threat of communism and second, it established a method of industrial management.[79] In World War II, there was a command economy, and wage and price control was influenced by Washington. The US economy prospered from the war and industrial production was almost quadrupled. Military spending was considered to be the main reason for America's rise from the depression and constant security threats throughout the post-war period maintained heavy investment of public funds in the electronic industry, aircraft industry and information technology.

However, this post-war boom on both sides of the Atlantic was about to come to an abrupt end. In the UK, 70 million days were lost to industrial disputes between 1970 and 1974 and effectively capsized the Heath administration. The proud post-war economic record of high unemployment, low inflation, and steady growth foundered with the OPEC price rise and subsequent international economic crisis. The rise in oil prices, combined with the financial and social disaster that was Vietnam, meant that the US share of global output slumped from 38% in 1970 to 25% just 10 years on.

1975 Onward: The Response

Towards the late 1970s, the UK was still oriented toward a benevolent social policy. The 1977 Housing Act extended the duties of local authorities with regards to the housing of the homeless and the Inner Urban Areas Act designated districts of deprivation for special treatment. That said, the international and domestic slump was facilitating change in the political and economic ethos in both the US and the UK. In the UK, Keynesian social democracy was coming under huge pressure from a group of politicians and business leaders whose faith in free market economics was gaining credibility among the right wing political parties and their acolytes. With the strained economic climate, these so-called neoliberals sought sanctuary, not in government control and regulation, but in the vagaries of the free market. The public sector was becoming a battleground for predatory private interests and social democracy was under attack from what was effectively a new variant on social Darwinism.

It was a time of manifest political and social change with the UK losing its historic identity as a protestant nation as church numbers fell rapidly after 1970. The labor movement was being transformed both by circumstances and by the incumbent administration as Callaghan's 1976 speech to the party conference accepted the inevitability of monetarism (and, indeed, the intervention of the IMF) and the existence of a 'natural' rate of unemployment. In the UK in the 1970s, declining productivity and slower economic growth reduced tax revenue, whilst rising unemployment continued to increase the demand for welfare. Like all good conservatives, Margaret Thatcher, the leader of the Conservative Party, reacted by calling on the precepts of the past as she heralded the by-now standard return to Victorian values.

Such forces as the women's movement, affirmative action and the sexual revolution fed a conservative backlash and the end of the 1970s found a disorientated class of conservatives in both the UK and the US, desperate to bring back the glories of a half-remembered era of nostalgic prosperity. So what were these neoliberals proposing that could be so effective at addressing the ills of the western world?

The Neoliberals and the Free Market

In post-war Britain, memories of wartime solidarity had faded fast and communitarian ties grew feeble as the hedonism of the individual returned with a vengeance. Something happened in the US and the UK that was not happening worldwide. Technological, social and economic changes arose that undermined the post-war democratic consensus and national identities reasserted themselves. Margaret Thatcher mined a feeling of populist, radical and anti-European nationalism and found that people seemed to agree with her assertion that there had been too much emphasis on class and not enough emphasis on the solidarity of nationhood. Until the late 1970s, the UK had shared a social democratic political ethos with its European partners but this was about to change. The economic climate deteriorated and the neoliberal New Right believed that they could address the failures of social democracy.

The major goal of the neoliberals was to separate governments from the economic fluctuations that result from the judgment of voters; to allow this Anglo-American singularity of the free market unparalleled importance in economic and political deci-sion making.[80] Neoliberalism presented itself as a theory but was actually a staid set of prescriptions designed to protect wealth and, more particularly, those who have it.

They championed economic liberalism and celebrated economic freedom. Much of the theory was based on the work of Milton Friedman who had made free market fundamentalism available and acceptable to a mass audience by focusing on its ability to liberate people and introduce prosperity. Supply-side economics was the new US panacea for political and social ills and Arthur Laffer, Jude Wanniski and George Gilder preached the benefits of their new theoretical perspective with no little zeal. However, the more discerning observer would have noted that this per-spective was not actually new being as it was essentially a simulation of simple trickle down economics.

The basic premise relied on heavy tax cuts that would encourage growth to soar. Inflation would decline and saving rates would rise without having to slash federal spending or endure a recession. The supply-side mantra stated that tax savings would be ploughed back into the production of job-creating activities. A more cynical commentator might suggest that corporations would simply use any extra capital as leverage to acquire other companies or increase their own profits at the expense of the consumers who were supposed to bear the fruit of these lowered costs. This theory was very much a staple of early 'Reaganomics' and supported the belief that only large corporations could revitalize the flagging US economy. Indeed, Reagan embraced Arthur Laffer and the supply-side acolytes and, despite evidence that he did not fully understand the theory,[81] he was convinced that this would be the way to get the US economy back on its feet. It is possible that under-standing the theory was actually less important than having a theory that embraced low taxes, regardless of what form it would take. In a display of rhetoric not strong on humility, these policies were discussed by Laffer's disciples as not only the savior of an economic decline but also the moral decline. Supply-side would also apparently bring people closer to God.[82]

In the UK, this 'unrevolutionary' turn of political events was somewhat inevitable, given that parliamentary absolutism rather than power sharing or coalition building lie at the heart of the political traditions of this country. Indeed Marquand[78] noted that parliamentary absolutism gave birth to neoliberalism. The neoliberals supported policies that included the privatization of public sector assets, tax cuts across the board, the disempowerment of trade unions and the introduction of free market economics into as many areas of modern life as was possible. This meant establishing government deregulation as a defining ethos because only by removing the government's power to intervene in business could free markets truly be 'free'. State planning and power had to be dismantled, cuts had to be made in welfare programmes and policies aimed towards full employment had to be abandoned.

The History and 'Naturalness' of Weak Government

The traditional raison d'être of a government is to protect its citizens from insecurity. However, the neoliberal revolution was at odds with this precept. For their utopia of a market-driven economy to be realized, government control and regulation had to be curbed. The construction of a free market depends on trade unions and any sense of collective power being destroyed or marginalized. That way employment rights and regulations can be made more flexible and hence amenable to corporate interests. This means an increase in part time and temporary work at the expense of traditional jobs and the associated job security. Governments were considered by the neoliberals to be overly intrusive. In the very business interests that would make nations strong and robust, government could only hurt stability and economic growth. Government was represented by these economic revolutionaries as obscure and inefficient, whereas private capital was able to bring clarity and efficiency towards the management of an economy.

One of the arguments advanced by many neoliberals was that a movement towards neoliberal precepts represented a 'natural' progression that was anchored in the 'natural' instincts of man to seek to acquire and maintain wealth and status. This kind of social Darwinism had been given a biological context in the previous century. Traditional liberal sentiments like community and government control were seen to be holding countries and citizens back from maximizing their inherent financial potential and free markets were the natural development that provided such opportunities.

Somewhere near the base of such logic usually exists the behaviour of nature and the hierarchical behaviour of chimps has been appropriated on more than one occasion to explain human misery and avarice. Nature is represented by the savage and selfish behaviour of our nearest ancestors and this portrayal of nature has been called on by a number of commentators to justify the self-serving structure of economic systems. If chimps could talk they would have hired Max Clifford (prominent UK public relations guru for those fortunate enough not to have encountered his work) by now because they need some very serious PR work. The logic goes something like this: animals like chimps inevitably show competitive social hierarchies and pecking orders and so humans justify market-led dominance and inequality by looking at the parallels in nature. If the 'survival of the fittest' happens in nature then it must right? Well no. For a start these chimps do not inevitably show competitive dominance hierarchies and different forms of social organization are possible among our closest relatives. Second, and perhaps more important, no matter how 'bright' these creatures are they are still not nearly as bright as human beings. The dullest humans are more cogent than the Stephen Hawking of the chimp world. So bearing this in mind, why do so many people read so much importance into the behaviour of a group of monkeys? Like the bible, biology is dipped in to justify different types of human behaviour and usually with similar unfailing inaccuracy.

Anyway I digress. This was not the first time that free market fundamentalism had gained momentum and history is instructive as to the consequences of such an economic outlook. However, historical lessons can be presented in a number of ways. Mid-nineteenth century England experienced a far-reaching social engineering experiment. Economic development was freed from social and political control and a free market was constructed in order to action such freedom and break up smaller, community-based markets.[80] This was not a natural occurrence as many free market apologists have argued, rather it relied on massive state intervention in order to transfer common land into private property. This was actioned by a relatively small group of profoundly wealthy industrialists/politicians whose political remit had been secured by a relatively disenfranchised population with few viable political alternatives. The repeal of the Corn Laws and the Poor Law Act in 1834 meant that individuals were solely responsible for their own welfare and those who failed were brutally stigmatized and, as mentioned earlier, forced into the workhouse.

Not until the creation of the Labour Party and extended suffrage were people able to restrain this project in such a way that the improvements in social policy touched upon earlier were enacted. Hence, this nineteenth century free market fundamentalism did not occur by chance as some natural and inevitable process but took the considerable efforts of the political classes to completely remodel society to their advantage. This way they could exploit recent technological, agricultural and industrial innovations. For the vast majority of the population, the process was about as natural as it is for an untouched chess piece to move on a board since they had no say in the matter. Their natural instincts were neither embraced nor denied since they were simply powerless.

Theories that posit markets as machines tend to neglect the fact that they are human inventions but the neoliberals wanted to create an arena where they were discussed as inevitable progressions rather than political alternatives. Certainly, momentum and time help such an acceptance of these 'natural' processes. The longer people live with institutions like markets, the more we begin to know ourselves through the precepts of these markets and then the market does come to seem natural. Society provides the cues that we use to interpret our thoughts and those of others and it is easy for people to come to understand themselves through what their culture tells them they are. It is easy to believe that whatever way that a society has been constructed has been the direct result of natural human needs and desires and that any resultant flaws are human flaws rather than those of social institutions.[83] The real problem that the neoliberals faced was reinstituting market fundamentalism in the first place. However, towards the end of the 1970s, the deteriorating social and economic experience in the US and the UK provided the perfect opportunity and the New Right seized the initiative.

The Realities of New Right Ideology

The realities of the neoliberal experiment differed considerably from the rhetoric and even the most dogged supply-siders would struggle to justify some of the outcomes. In the US, state enterprises worth around $180 billion were sold to the private sector in the 1980s. The election of Margaret Thatcher's conservatives in 1979 and Ronald Reagan's republicans in 1980 gave political voice to the new right revolutionaries and a programme of marginalization of trade unions and local authorities, privatization of state enterprises and the imposition of market logic on the public sector proceeded apace in both the UK and the US. The supposed naturalness of market capitalism was illustrated by massive state interventions pushed through by ruthless centralized bureaucracies.

The language of individual rights became prominent and such concepts as civic responsibility and mutual obligations were traded in for a focus on individual wealth acquisition. Such a change meant that power could swiftly move from the political sphere to the private economy with governments less able and willing to make decisions about public investment, employment and the control of resources.

This market logic would lead directly and indirectly to social breakdown on a genuinely significant scale with almost all areas of society affected. This included the cohesion of the family unit, financial strain and inequality, occupational rights and roles, public representation, crime, health, mental health and alienation amongst others. Social democracy was unceremoniously ejected and the UK and the US became the main repositories for these economic and social changes. Choice, and the freedom to choose, was marketed as the principal benefit of such an approach and conservatives and republicans sold (and continue to sell) their agenda on the basis that people were being empowered by their policies. This famously conservative 'right to choose' is one of the great right wing maxims, the right of every single right-minded citizen and when portrayed in this light it sounded like a pretty good deal.

However, at the risk of being a prophet of the obvious, not everyone had the same right to choose since different groups of people had varying political, economic and material resources. Market fundamentalism leads inexorably to greater differentials in this freedom of choice as people choose within their structural contexts, dictated by powers beyond their influence. As such, the concept of choice needs to be treated very carefully. The right to choose which hospital to take your child to or which school they are educated in has been discussed by the new right as one of the great civilizing forces in modern western society, free market economics the saviour that can bring this choice to everyone. It has been located at the heart of people's social and economic desires when actually what most people want are good schools and good hospitals universally so that they know that their local amenities are capable of providing the service they deserve. Choice only becomes an issue when mismanagement, economic disparities and under-funding result in health and education options that are markedly substandard. Rather than free market fundamentalism introducing a mythical choice-induced standard of excellence, it further perpetuates economic disparities between those who have 'choice' and those who do not. Material disadvantage eliminates much of the choice that most people are supposed to have and the political discourses of a liberal capitalist system preserves the illusion that those who make the wrong choices are responsible for their own misfortune. Their failure is not sending their children to private school or not choosing to buy their own home or have private health care plans.

Most liberal individualist and free market acolytes repudiate the fact that people have duties beyond paying (little) taxes and obeying the law. As a member of a new right society, this was the extent of our duties and Margaret Thatcher even went so far as to say that there was no such thing as society, so little did she believe in civic responsibility. Indeed liberal individualism can actually be defined by rights against the community. Citizenship concerns such values as loyalty, public duties and obligation; it does not focus on rights and so is antithetical to the new right. The value of being a citizen in society was under grave threat.

So What Actually Happened in the US During the 1980s?

At the beginning of the 1980s, political transformation in both the US and the UK ushered in widespread social and economic changes that have since been maintained by successive administrations. As mentioned, these changes were very specific to these countries.[78] Only in the 1980s and 1990s had the free market become the dominant social institution and the incorporation of free markets into the daily polity encouraged new inequalities in income, wealth, access to work and quality of life.[80]

As with Thatcher in the UK, politics in the US came to be dominated by a single political figure, a former Hollywood movie star and state governor of California. Ronald Reagan and his supporters positioned themselves as people who wanted to get their country back on the right track by returning America to its spiritual roots.

In the 1970s, many professional's wages barely kept up with inflation. Financing for the unemployment insurance system deteriorated and state reserves became exhausted. At the turn of the 1980s, voters agreed with Reagan that the economy had been mismanaged, although that did not necessarily mean that there was a significant consensus for right wing issues like pro-lifeism and the drastic cutting of welfare programmes that became staples of the administration. Reaganites used the rhetoric of an America that was adrift at sea, shorn of its bearings; a country that could only be saved by revisiting the kind of political choices that had made it great in the past. To Reagan, this meant a return to the ethos of Calvin Coolidge's ultra-conservative administration of the 1920s. In the US, like the UK, there was a deep sense of frustration combined with a series of political, economic and, in the case of the US, military failures that had struck at the nation's sense of itself. Interest rates reached 21%, the highest they had been since the civil war over 100 years earlier and the public failure of the Carter administration to secure a release for the American hostages in Iran had culminated in a need for change.

Prior to 1980, a small group of profoundly rich Californians had decided that Ronald Reagan was their man and resolved to place him in the White House via the governorship of California. This way the White House could be converted into a shrine to conservatism that would promote the kind of economic and social policies that these businessmen subscribed to. Reagan represented these self-made men, rugged individualists who believed that their interests were synonymous with the interests of America. For such conservatives, good government meant no government, a throwback to this ethos of the 1920s. With Reagan's emergence, many disaffected groups found a counterpoint around which to rally against years of civil disobedience, unpatriotic anti-Vietnam sentiment and student rallies.

Whilst generating monumental ideological vigor, Reagan showed that he was a conservative of a new breed, a consumer rather than a preserver, and came to dominate his era as such. In his inaugural address, Reagan set out his political stall when he said that government was not the solution but the problem that was driving America's problems. He emphasized that he was on the side of property, the family and the flag, not all of which he proved in the following 8 years. Moreover he was a crucial driving force behind the celebration of the acquisition of personal wealth.

Reagan the man had only a passing acquaintance with some of the most important policy decisions of his administration[81] and he took delegation to unprecedented levels in his determination to focus himself on the handful of issues that interested him. These included destroying jobs, increasing social inequality and the national deficit, and castigating welfare recipients. When time permitted, he also squeezed in the destruction of the morale and status of public servants. Many sources have confirmed that he liked to communicate in anecdotes rather than policy formulations and some of his own officials described him as intellectually lazy and 'without a constant curiosity'.[84] However he was not without political nous. He was particularly adept at presenting himself as the nice guy surrounded by unpleasant autocrats and bureaucrats, often distancing himself from some of his administration's more outlandish policy decisions like propping up brutal dictatorships, ravaging his own countryside (although his claim that 80% of the nation's air pollution problems having been caused by chemicals released by trees suggested that this was more out of ignorance than malice) and creating mammoth social inequality through favouring the wealthy.

In 1981, Reagan produced for Congress the most wildly inaccurate budget in US history. It suggested a balanced national budget over the next 3 years, a claim made impossible by the increase in military expenditure during this time. The money spent on the military jumped from $182 billion in 1982 to $216 billion only a year later. Previous military build-ups happened during strong commercial booms, whereas this one happened because it was what the administration wanted, regardless of the condition of the economy, which happened to be in a severe recession. Reagan uncoupled the age-old relationship between tax and social policy as he sought his impossible dream of heavy tax cuts and high increases in military spending but an inevitable fiscal crisis developed as the national debt plummeted out of control.

Generally speaking, he showed little interest, indeed a degree of contempt, for the political machinations of high office and his role in the Iran-Contra saga highlighted this as well as anything during his regime. He specifically ordered that information be held from US congressional oversight committees and the fact that the CIA were specifically banned from supporting the contras by dint of a definitive legal act passed by the House of Representatives meant little to the Reagan administration.[81]

Deregulation Fever

Reagan's popularity increased hugely in the early 1980s as a result of his facing down the air traffic controller's strike, by surviving his shooting and the equanimity of the remarks associated with both the incident and his recovery. This kind of popularity inevitably awards politicians legislative leeway and Reagan took full advantage. His policies themselves could best be described as an amalgam of ideas culled from such venerable sources as neoconservatism, fundamentalism and the good, old fashioned back to basics backlash against any remotely progressive civil liberties. Essentially, it was social Darwinism and he represented the many constituents who felt that they had lost something in Vietnam and were continuing to lose as a result of civil rights pressures.

In Reagan's America, there was little need for such sources of social security as housing assistance or the minimum wage since the growing disparity between the haves and the have-nots was simply a result of a difference in application between the two groups. This could be addressed by hard work on the part of the less fortunate. To reduce a growing national deficit, his administration reduced funding for job training and tried to eliminate the Trade Adjustment Act benefits, which allowed compensation and retraining of workers who lost jobs as a result of foreign imports.

In 1987, the US congress passed the Interstate Commerce Act, which allowed the federal government to regulate private interests when they considered them to be contrary to the public good. However, such legislation, while appearing to many as a reasonable representation of the interests of the electorate, was attacked ferociously by the Reagan administration. This formed part of Reagan's 'war on regulation', with the likes of occupational health legislation, the Consumer Product Safety Commission and the Environmental Protection Agency all experiencing the effects of this deregulatory fever. Indeed James Millar III, his new chairman of the Federal Trade Commission noted that his agency needed to 'stop protecting consumers against false advertising and defective products'.[81] God forbid such outrageous overprotection should be forced on the American citizens.

Reagan, however, was always the friend of corporate America and much of his deregulation was aimed at allowing American business to operate in an environment most conducive to profit generation, although not necessarily with great consideration to the people of America who were exposed to the downside of such deregulation. For instance, his deregulation initiatives spread to the Federal Communications Commission and led to their dropping such pesky regulations as those which meant that broadcasters had to devote a minimum amount of airtime to news and public service programmes. The FCC also increased the amount of advertising that a station could run in an hour. The number of stations that a company could own was increased from five to twelve, thus encouraging the development of media and television monopolies. Inevitably this had a knock on effect for the kind of programming and news content displayed by such stations and 'off message' content would suffer as a result of corporate influence. The FCC's long standing fairness doctrine, which required balanced presentation of a public issue, was also abandoned, further reducing the public service element of telebroadcasting.

The Reagan administration's most extensive deregulation activities related to the market for corporate control and following relaxation of the antitrust laws, a flurry of financial mergers took off. Company 'efficiency' became the byword as hawks in the finance industry bought firms, broke them into component parts for sale and radically decreased the workforce in order to prompt savings. The often drastic social effects of such drives for efficiency were not at the top of the industrial agenda. Buyers would often borrow heavily to make such acquisitions and repayment and profit was funded by whatever drives towards efficiency were possible. We were introduced to the benefits of 'flexibility' as companies sought to achieve this by making extended use of temporary and contract workers, although it was not always clear how the removal of occupational predictability and security increased flexibility for employees. The 1980s was an era of increased overtime and reductions in vacations, rest periods and time off. For white collar workers, large scale lay-offs and a more cutthroat job environment led to a need to devote greater time and resources to the working environment, whereas for low-wage workers, sweatshops appeared with Victorian-style working conditions.[85] The reaction of the governments in the US and the UK was to further erode protection for employees as well as conspicuously fail to enforce existing work regulations.

The nature of the balance between job security for workers and increased efficiency and productivity for corporations took a huge swing towards corporations and many people went from working in a secure and content environment to living lives where unpredictable income was the norm. Such a lack of security in their work left employees feeling more inclined to address their own interests and could conceivably have contributed to a greater sense of isolation.[81]

Deregulation in the stock market brought back investors. Reduced commissions and the growth in computers allowed institutions to trade in greater volumes than had previously been possible. This led to greater volatility in the stock market and hundreds of companies were subjected to acquisition or mergers with experts (and future guests in US Penitentiaries as a result of insider trading) like Ivan Boesky and Michael Milken able to earn obscene commissions. Financial safeguards that had existed since the great crash of 1929 were modified or removed completely by the Reagan administration.

If an administration places such emphasis on corporate deregulation and the privatization of public services, the path is inevitably open for avaristic public officials to exploit their positions for personal gain and the Reagan administration was marred by a particularly high number of public scandals involving officials cashing in on their public positions. Bribes, government contracts, influence peddling and fraud were rife and by May 1985 there were 131 separate investigations pending against a number of the defense departments' most important contractors.[81] It would be naïve to suggest that such events had not occurred in previous administrations but it is reasonable to conclude that it became endemic in the US in the 1980s and Reagan's administration was simply the worst in history for such crimes. A particularly forceful revolving door policy meant that government procurement officials very quickly became private weapons contract consultants. The Housing and Urban Development Department became a particularly nefarious source of exploitation, a vehicle for the politically powerful and wealthy to exploit low income housing programmes that were originally intended to aid the poor.

Tax, Income Redistribution and the 'W word'

If there was one defining political principle of the Reagan administration, and probably the man himself, it would be that of tax cuts. Ever the corporate panderer, Reagan was drawn to tax cuts like few politicians before him and his administration spearheaded the charge for $142 billion in tax cuts for corporations in the first 5 years. This was the first step in a reduction programme designed to encourage capital investment and which would eventually see America exhibit the lowest corporate taxes of any major industrialized country.[82] His 1983 budget included a 15% drop in education funding (on top of inflation erosion) and a drop in funding for such obvious 'non-essentials' as housing and urban development, welfare payments and food stamps. He implemented huge income tax reductions under the aegis of encouraging consumer spending and sought to eliminate job training programmes. This is particularly significant since some 2 million industrial jobs disappeared during the 1980s, many of them in areas with high concentrations of black workers. The burden of tax, usually through stealth and indirect taxes, moved to the less wealthy, many of whom worked in manufacturing and so were suffering declines in the values of their real wages during this time.

Reagan used his compliant congress to institute the most significant income redistribution since the 1930s only this time in the opposite direction to Roosevelt's

New Deal policies. Resources were transferred from the public sector to the private sector and corporate profits were the benchmark of an administration that had placed its faith in big business making America great again. And what is more likely to interfere with corporate profit than providing aid to the needy? Welfare has long been the enemy of rank and file conservatives but it became an especially dirty word in the political lexicon of the 1980s. In a country with little real union power, the slashing of social programmes reinstated the terror of being jobless for those with and without jobs. To attract corporate investment, state governments were under pressure to lower taxes and hence benefit levels.

Federal policies had always traditionally promoted economic and social mobility but deregulation, the disparagement of government and the slashing of taxes and welfare had profound effects on a significant proportion of the American public. The black poor and women suffered particularly as a result of Reagan's cutbacks and were disproportionately represented on programmes like the Aid to Families with Dependent Children (AFDC, which has dropped around 40% in real terms between 1970 and 1995[79]), food stamps, federally subsidized daycare, Medicaid, family planning and legal aid.

The American middle class shrunk and a gulf developed between the good life enjoyed by a select few and the life of social helplessness, poverty and resignation experienced by many. Economic disparity grew dramatically during the 1980s and between 1979 and 1997, the after-tax income of the poorest 20% of US households decreased by $100, whereas the top 1% of households enjoyed a 157% after-tax income increase.[86] Although the electronics industry was booming in Silicon valley, many industries were declining. In factory and farm communities, the unemployment was twice that of the national average and many were forced to take minimum wage jobs without health insurance or other benefits that they had previously enjoyed. In the Midwest, soup kitchens appeared for the first time since the 1930s. In the rustbelt states, poverty became endemic and with it the usual partners in crime; family abuse, violence, crime and divorce and family separations were commonplace as men traveled around the country in search of work.

The Culture of America in the 1980s

A cursory glance towards the American film industry during this time tells a familiar story and one which complimented the prevailing political ethos. It was common for Hollywood to chart the struggles of individuals against large, complex and often unspecified enemies and such insularity provided a new impetus to the individualism that was already a bedrock of American culture. The growing time spent on technology-based leisure pursuits like television and video added to this impetus and by the end of the 1980s American people spent, on average, seven hours watching television in a given day. Television advertising revenue had reached $23 billion annually by 1990. The considerable effects of this growth in television advertising are discussed in the next chapter.

It was an era when entertainment constituted watching outrageously wealthy families squabble over oil rights or who owned a given stable of horses and Dynasty and Dallas emerged as national and international phenomena. Incredible decadence became the context for popular entertainment. It was during this decade that the 'Yuppie' was born; the young urban professionals preoccupied with the generation of the wealth and income necessary to move towards the kind of lifestyle enjoyed by Bobby Ewing and Blake Carrington. It also allowed them to keep up with the latest consumer trends that increased television advertizing regularly beamed into their front rooms. It was the decade where credit card spending (and credit card debt) doubled. Between 1980 and 1988, US credit card spending went from $205 billion to $397 billion as the number of malls and shopping centers in America increased by two thirds.

There was an enormous increase in religious broadcasters moving into the political forum during the 1980s and evangelical preachers came to enjoy unprecedented access to the president. Such Christian fundamentalism was embraced by Reagan who had previously informed the Californian State Senate in 1971[87] that his personal religious crusade was based on Ezekiel. The Soviets became Gog, the nation that would lead all others towards darkness and he had few qualms about discussing the Soviet Union as the focus of evil in the modern world (a precursor to George W. Bush's 'axis of evil', a category that appears to contain anyone he does not like, be it Saddam Hussein, Osamah Bin Laden, the Taleban and the guy from catering who burnt his toast this morning).

Televangelists were conservative, they believed in embracing the power of money and they sought to amalgamate the influence of religion, entertainment and patriotism into one narrow-minded and hypocritical package. Some, like George Gilder, were even able to state that free-enterprise capitalism could unleash a religiously inspired spirit of benevolence, although it would not always be easy to square such spiritual growth with the stricter, communitarian teachings of the bible. In a country where 70% of citizens believe in the devil (as opposed to 30% in UK, 20% in France and 12% in Sweden),[87] the moral majority were able to come to the fore and show just how much power a well-organized, religiously militant and intolerant minority could have over the political process. Only a series of ridiculous sex scandals involving the leaders of the movement managed to throw them off course but for a period their ethically questionable political campaigns ruined the careers of a number of honest politicians.

The End of Reagan

As with Thatcher in the UK, Reagan managed to break the inflation spiral on the back of the jobless and one of his overriding achievements was to make a notoriously inert, centrist consensus like the US political body accommodate change so quickly. He also helped to effect a large scale change in the attitudes of the public and many millions of American citizens bought into the Reagan vision of hope and optimism. His appeals focused on the nostalgia of a long forgotten time when complex national problems had easy solutions. He helped to generate a change in public attitudes to wealth and success, and personal greed and glory were elevated to the status of dominant virtues.

Reagan indulged big business to an unprecedented level. He preached deregulation, created an ethos that denigrated public service and allowed US business to become less competitive as investment in education and advanced technologies fell at the sword of short-termism. His administration was weakened by scandal and ethical ambiguity with the Iran Contra affair and the conduct of such high profile colleagues like Michael Deaver and Ed Meese, but never to the extent that he was in real political chaos.

As he closed his second term, he sanctimoniously intoned that 'we meant to change a nation, instead we changed a world' and that 'we've done our part'. To the end he was probably not aware of the extent of the damage he had caused to the social fabric of America and Robert Wright of the New Republic described the final years of his administration as 'a battle for the soul of a man who was virtually brain dead'.[84]

What Were the Results of These Changes in the US?

The old saying goes that 'it is cheaper to feed the child than to jail the man' but such wisdom was not in vogue in the US in the 1980s. The phrase could have been more appropriately amended to 'it is cheaper to feed the child than jail the man but who cares?' 1989 found the US with half of its black children living in poverty and with the highest divorce rate in the world. One in five children in the US lived with a single parent and that parent was far more likely to work than not, leaving a huge number of children unsupervised.

As with all societies where social policies favour the wealthy (and hence exhibit high inequality) the children generally show lower levels of educational achievements. It usually takes some years for the true effects of the social policies of an administration to seep through into the culture as a whole and these effects do not make pleasant reading for Reagan enthusiasts (although to be fair such enthusiasts are probably not overly perturbed by virtue of being Reagan enthusiasts). In 1999, the US census bureau stated that the poverty rate was 29% in the US among households headed by a woman. About 12.1 million children were 'poor' by federal standards and this represented 17% of the nation's children.[88] However, the census bureau figures do not take into account medication, health, laundry, transport and childcare and if they did so then a further 17% of the population would be considered to be living in poverty. Other sources have suggested that over 31 million Americans live below the poverty line with 41% of those having less than half the official income of the poverty line.[89] Hunger is increasingly a problem for poor women and children in the US[89] and in recent years UNICEF showed that 9 million US children suffered from malnutrition.

Regarding inequality in wages, 1960 found the average corporate chief executive making 41 times the average worker but, as a result of the Reagan administration and subsequent administration's redistributive policies, the figure stood at 115 times the average worker in 1999. Moreover, between the late 1970s and the late 1990s, the average income for US families in the bottom fifth of the income scale fell by 5%, whereas that of the top fifth rose by 33%[88] and congressional efforts to increase a declining federal minimum wage have been unsuccessful.

The period between 1979 and 1982 saw massive federal budget deficits and widespread plant closings led to the dislocation of millions of workers.[90] Indeed, in the five year period up to 1984, 11.5 million workers lost their jobs because of plant shut downs, relocations or abolished jobs. The new jobs that have been created in the US economy in recent years have tended to be low-level, poorly paid and often part-time or temporary with few, if any, benefits. More than half of the 8 million jobs created between 1979 and 1984 paid less than $7000 a year.[90] Of the jobs with the greatest growth, 74% are considered to pay less than a livable wage and 46% pay less than half of what is considered to be a livable wage.[88] These jobs have tended to be in the service domain, particularly fast-food and retail. Such stunning progress is not 'growth' as we traditionally understand it but a direct result of allowing corporations greater 'flexibility' and 'freedom' at the expense of the quality of life of the general public. Indeed, the largest groups of poor people in the US are not those on welfare but the working poor[88] and work often fails to protect many people from financial insecurity and deprivation. American workers now work more hours per year than any other industrialized nation but with fewer sources of essential support like parental leave and subsidized childcare.[89]

Workers who participate in adjustment programmes and who complete training programmes tend to have considerably less unemployment and lower loss of income (and hence less social and personal difficulties associated with job loss) but the provision of satisfactory advanced notice of job termination and the active participation in readjustment programmes tends to be the exception to the rule.[90] During 1983 and 1984, 55% of blue collar workers and 44% of white collar workers received either no notice or up to 14 days notice and, perhaps unsurprisingly, the 1985 Secretary of Labor's task force on economic adjustment and worker dislocation concluded that companies in the private sector made inadequate effort to help their displaced employees. The effort was so inadequate that the 1986 report of the Congressional Office of Technology noted that adjustment and training programmes met the needs of only 5% of workers who were displaced.[90]

The need for employers to provide advance notice of plant closing, making them subscribe to plant closing guidelines and providing targeted assistance to maintain income and health benefits to the affected communities is crucial but regulation for this should contain a political impetus with the legislation coming from state level. However, as the states compete for new business, the more flexibility that they offer firms with regard to their workforce, the more likely they are to secure business in their area. With a government seemingly allergic to any kind of federal initiatives to protect their workers, many people suffered as a result of the closure of plants and discontinuation of jobs. By contrast, continental European worker adjustment programmes generally include wage subsidies, relocation assistance, income maintenance beyond unemployment insurance benefits, advance notice, job training and job creation provisions as well as support from the government for early retirement. Reagan, ever keen to exhibit his support for the business community, showed his charitable side by vetoing a 1988 bill because it required a 60 day advance notice for firms with 100 or more employees.[90]

Health care has also suffered and by the end of the 1990s, a WHO analysis ranked the US 37th in the world overall with regard to its standard of health care. Crime figures told a story of profound racial divides in the allocation of resources. A black male was four times more likely to go to prison than a black South African during apartheid and by 1992 a quarter of black males in their twenties were either in prison, on parole or on probation compared to one in sixteen white males.[76] As such, the 1992 Los Angeles riots should not have come as a complete surprise to the US government.

If we summarize the figures between the start and the end of the 1980s, the fruition of Reaganite policies could proudly boast of an extra 22% of children in poverty, a 10% increase in the juvenile custody rate and an 11% increase in the rates of violent deaths of children aged between 15 and 19 years old.[76]

So What Actually Happened in the UK During the 1980s?

As late as 1975, progressive legislation in the UK was still being directed towards those with the greatest needs. Acts were passed that placed all social insurance benefits on an earnings-related basis, provided an inflation-proof, single-rate, earnings-related pension and provided mothers with an inflation-proof weekly payment for all children, with additional benefits for single mothers. However, only five years later a contrast in social policy led to an Education Act that limited free school meals, relaxed the school's obligations to provide milk and completely removed the obligation to provide nursery education. The Social Security Act removed the link between benefits and earnings and cut the uprating of benefits. The Employment Act banned secondary picketing by trades union, limited to six the number of people on a picket line and introduced trade union ballots and codes of practice. So what happened in the intervening five years?

Of all the European right wing parties in the late 1970s, the UK Conservative Party became, by some distance, the most dogmatic. With a financial approach that could be alternately referred to as monetarism, neoliberalism or just plain Thatcherism, it was heavily influenced by the work of Milton Friedman, a right wing economist who believed that his theory straddled the boundary between science and faith. Indeed, such quaisi-religious zealotry was shared by many free market liberals. Thatcherism itself was a dogma and as such was less susceptible to reflection than a more typical political movement but the chronic lack of credible political opposition during the time allowed the Thatcher ideologues great freedom to experiment with free market fundamentalism and the UK economy.[91] Much like

Reagan's revolution across the Atlantic, Thatcherism ensconced the virtues of enterprise culture, deregulation and limited state control wherever possible. This also meant the diminution of the capacities of trades union through reform, rapaciously promoting capital ownership and, of course, slashing taxes. Privatization was a bedrock of the Thatcherite approach not only because it placed public services in the hands of private corporations but because it curbed union power within these services and it was not unusual for her administration to use the process of privatization to reward its wealthy supporters.

Although Thatcher purported to the role of demagogue for the reintroduction of Victorian values, her political ethos actually had surprisingly little in common with these values that she held so dear.[92] The Thatcher concept of society was that it simply did not exist. Thatcher was paradoxically devoted to the idea of a strong state and a free market. She wanted to introduce market logic into every area of British politics and The 1988 Education Act, with the introduction of the National Curriculum, attainment tests and league tables, served just such an example in the educational arena. While the purpose of the act was to make education at all levels accountable to its consumers, a chronic lack of investment and a 10%[92] reduction in public spending on schools between 1979 and 1986 meant that education inevitably failed to become a paragon of free market success.

Efficiency drives also led to the Thatcher administration reducing the number of civil servants by 23% and the Local Government Act in 1988 ensured that local government put most of their services out to private tender. Local democracy had already been wounded by the government's 1984 Rate Act, which had removed the power of local authorities to determine their own rate (tax) level. Although such centralization was rowing against the European tide, by limiting the power of local government she was able to limit the financial autonomy of Labour-controlled councils and hence levels of rates that she considered abominable.

Privatization and Public Spending

The privatization of council properties was one of Thatcher's great crusades and discounts on the financial value of properties and tax relief for mortgage interest repayments acted as inducements to buy. According to Thatcher, council estates were breeding grounds for crime, socialism, violence and general antisocial behaviour, and she saw private property ownership as the tool to combat the malcontents thrown up by such estates.[93] This formed the backbone of what she described in 1987 as 'their really big job to do on the inner cities'.

Reckless borrowing was encouraged, which led to inflation and a spate of repossessions and negative equity in the early 1990s as the property bubble burst. Such financial inducements were excellent for those who could afford their own properties but could be seen as a little unfair as they were part-funded by tax relief at the expense of the general public. Basically, if you could afford your own property then you were in business but otherwise you had to sit back and help your wealthier neighbour up the road by providing more money to help him afford his. Around £28 billion was raised by these sales and it proved to be the most profitable of all the privatizations, more so than British Telecom, Gas and Electricity. This privatization also meant that there were reduced funds available for housing development and those that were available tended to focus on more desirable areas. The by-product of this was the creation of 'sink estates', ghettoized areas of housing where people could not afford to buy their own properties.

In truth, the Thatcher administration would have privatized anything that moved in the 1980s and even floated the idea of ending public funding of the National Health Service until it became obvious that some public services were beyond even their reach. That is not to say that sweeping market reforms did not take place in the NHS. Doctors became isolated as the language of the market place seeped insidiously into professional care and practice. The success of these market reforms in health was debatable since, by December 1987, some 4,000 beds were closed because funds were running out towards the end of the financial year. Moreover, divisions appeared between fund-holding and non fund-holding GPs. A fundamental lack of funding was betrayed by government statistics from the same year, which showed that the UK spent 5.9% of its GDP in health care compared to 9.1% in France, 8.1% in Germany and 7.2% in Italy. Schemes such as 'Care in the Community' for mental health patients allowed the government to cut costs but often at the expense of vulnerable patients who required greater treatment.

British Telecom, British Steel, British Airways and Rolls Royce, as well as the airports and water companies, were all sold off. As was perhaps inevitable with privatized public utilities, employment reduced (from 8 million to 3 million) as streamlining and efficiency drives created shareholder savings.[93] Such policies were not always in the interest of the organization as the pensioning off of many skilled engineers by Railtrack led to one of the most poorly administered British companies in recent history.[92]

Tax and Inflation

As with Reagan's administration in the US, Thatcher inherited the problem of high inflation and broke this inflation by creating a deep recession. It was hardly the most subtle or most effective way to reduce inflation; bankrupting a raft of businesses and throwing millions of people out of work, but this was Thatcher's idea of the best solution.

The mini-boom initiated by the abolition of hire-purchase restrictions brought about a resumption in growth,[91] although much of this huge expansion in consumer and business credit was spent on foreign imports and UK manufacturing, like its partner in the US, suffered. Between 1986 and 1988, house prices shot up by 40% but the government failed to address this explosion in credit. This administration was utterly committed to lowering taxes and the continual lowering of the base rate and increases in indirect taxation (as in the US) was not sustainable. Nigel Lawson, the Chancellor of the Exchequer, lowered taxes at the height of this boom and it had the same effect as trying to control a fire by throwing petrol on it. Inflation took off to the tune of 10% in 1990 and, as touched upon earlier, the UK lapsed into the longest recession since before the Second World War. Rising interest rates led to a spate of bankruptcies and the unemployment that followed led to many experiencing mortgage arrears. Negative equity and repossessions became commonplace and the UK experienced one of the worst and most irresponsible economic slumps since the war. This, together with the introduction of the poll tax, a monument to Thatcher's unquenchable desire to redistribute tax incentives to the wealthy, led inexorably to the drawing to a close of the Thatcher regime.

Welfare and Social Security

If there was a defining political arena in which the Thatcher administration worked their magic then it was social welfare. At a time when dramatic reductions in public spending were used as one arm of the fight to control inflation, and modifications of national taxation were operating to redistribute tax benefits from the less wealthy to the more wealthy (and particularly to the very rich), one might think a reduction in social security spending somewhat inopportune. However, this administration cut the value of real social security benefits as well as the number of claimants and, in 1982, linked pensions to prices rather than earnings. Further, in 1988 the young became the target of the conservative penny pinchers as the right to unemployment benefit was withdrawn from 16–17 year olds. Thatcher and Norman Fowler even tried to end the 'social travesty' that was universal child benefit but, like their dreams of destroying the National Health Service, this proved to be a bridge too far.

Essentially, Thatcher believed that welfare itself was responsible for some of the social illness experienced by the country and that it had a tendency to militate against economic achievement. She also believed that it generated a dependency culture where people would settle for welfare rather than seek out employment. Fortuitously, this also coincided with her need to reduce taxes and public spending as much as humanly possible. The fundamental issue was that she could never understand why it should be the role of the state to improve people's lives and welfare joined local government and Europe as political concepts, which, on a good day, she found utterly distasteful. The irony of moving more and more people on to welfare as a result of free market-driven economic policies that created high interest rates, bankruptcies, unemployment and 'streamlined and efficient' company mergers failed to register. After all, like Reagan, she believed wholeheartedly in the responsibilities of the individual to their own welfare rather than to any notion of social dependency and citizenship consisted of nothing more than paying tax and not committing crime. Dependency on the state was the last thing that Thatcher wanted to encourage, unless of course you count the wealthier members of society who counted on the state for mortgage tax relief and income tax cuts.

In the 2 years between 1979 and 1981, between a fifth and a quarter of UK manufacturing was wiped out and widespread riots in Brixton, Liverpool,

Birmingham, Leeds and Bradford highlighted a marginalized section of the population whose desperation drove them onto the streets. Thatcher responded to such civil unrest with her now famous 'this lady's not for turning' speech at the 1980 Conservative Party Conference. Unemployment grew (and indeed peaked at 3.15 million later in the 1980s) but uninspired opposition from the Labor benches failed to make the conservatives pay and reelection beckoned.

Increasing unemployment, slashing social security and then blaming the newly unemployed for being dependent, whilst still getting reelected, was a trick that could only be pulled off by a government that had created an agenda for a specific section of the populous, namely the property-owning, financially solvent electorate from the South East of England. Indeed, traditional mass production manufacturing had become rationalized and resources were shifted from the North East to the Thames Valley.[78]

The Thatcher administration, buoyed by the North Sea oil supply and supported by the more prosperous South East of England, recruited the Rupert Murdoch press bandwagon. This was particularly true in the shape of The Sun, with its daily circulation of 4 million. Indeed there was very little opposition to Thatcherite policies in Fleet Street.[75] When Murdoch wanted to buy the Times and the Sunday Times in 1980, his bid (that should have been required reading for the monopolies commission) failed to come under scrutiny and such neglect allowed him to control more than one third of the British National news press, a factor that might have contributed to his rabid support of the Thatcher administration. This support, together with the drive towards home-ownership, allowed the conservatives to make inroads into much of the traditional Labour support base, a support that was struggling with an unelectable leadership.

Thatcher's concept of 'conviction politics' and her narrow vision for the UK led to the destruction of political and social institutions with medium and long-term consequences. For many, the failure of the 1984 miner's strike represented the last line of defense against the technological and economic upheavals of Thatcherism. The 1984 Trade Union Act removed legal immunity from strikes that were not approved by their members in secret ballot and Scargill's failure to call an NUM ballot and achieve the support of anywhere near a majority of his members for the strike (18,000 voted for the strike and 40,500 against) hamstrung the strikers from the beginning.[91] By the 1987 Labor conference, doyens of the old left like Tony Benn felt that socialism was now mentioned almost in apology with a nudge and a wink[94] as the Labor juggernaut leaned more and more to the right in search of electoral credibility.

Poverty and Inequality: The Legacy of Thatcher's Britain

The 1980s saw a movement from the manufacturing sector to the service sector with an increase in non-unionized, female labor. Efficiency probes and ruthless cost cutting led to profound changes in the civil service as tenure was removed and with it, effective opposition to the government from Whitehall. Having a job for life meant that civil servants could tell cabinet ministers the truth as opposed to being pliant and powerless followers of the government initiatives of the day.[95] The effective removal of this potential level of opposition suited Thatcher, as it has suited politicians since, with governments creating public service policy in search of electoral support.

The thirst for deregulation attacked the rights of those under the age of 21, a substantial number of whom were already compromised by the withdrawal of unemployment benefit. Pay and work conditions were deregulated for this demographic and teenagers and young adults were open to exploitation. It is not clear exactly why Thatcher so disparaged the working rights of younger adults in the UK save for the recognition that they hardly constituted her core electoral support and so could be sacrificed at the alter of public spending reductions. The young were not the only UK workers who suffered as a result of conservative employment policy. In 1990, EC directives were proposed that might give part-time and temporary workers the same rights as full-time staff, but they were dismissed by the government.

The casualization of labour gave way to fractured communities as people often had to travel to find temporary work without the previous benefits that they might have enjoyed. It led to considerable anguish, with unpredictability regarding the meeting of financial commitments. Such casualization was undoubtedly beneficial for employers as this flexibility allowed them to increase profits without having to retain a constant workforce. There were benefits but they came at a price and this price was paid by employees and their communities. The traditional family declined during Thatcher's tenure with one parent families increasing from 12% in 1979 to 21% in 1992 and while such figures cannot be laid solely at the door of employment policy, such policy contributed significantly.

Although many conservatives questioned the folly of the exclusive reliance on the market to regulate all aspects of UK political life,[91] Thatcher's insistence on such logic led to huge transformations in almost every domain of her mythical society. There was an upsurge in poverty driven by the tripling of unemployment to over 3 million and the number of completely workless British households went from 6.5% in 1975 to 19.1% in 1994.[80]

That Thatcher saw the relative wealth of the electorate as none of the government's business did not bode well for those in the lower portions of the financial spectrum and unsurprisingly, an overwhelming majority were considerably worse off than they had been before Thatcher came to power. The average real income of the bottom 10% of the population fell by 14% between 1979 and 1991 while that of the richest 10% rose by a whopping 51%.[78] During the same time period, the number of people living on an income of lower than 40% of the national average increased fivefold to 7.7 m. Insufficient investment in new housing, the mauling of housing benefits and massive mortgage subsidies to wealthier citizens meant that the number of households considered as homeless grew from 57,000 to 127,000 under Thatcher,[91] although even this increase was a considerable underestimation as it did not include those sleeping rough. Only rabid neoliberals fail to understand that homelessness results not from the personal inadequacies of the homeless but from, among other things, a real shortage of decent homes at affordable prices and the necessary investment was simply absent. One effect of the Care in the Community programme was the unsupervised release onto the streets of many people with psychiatric disorders and this contributed to the figures above. A failure to appreciate that not all of the patients had personal communities to provide for their needs was irrelevant to Thatcher as her vacuous understanding of the needs of mental health patients suited her desire to slash public service funding. Thatcher's contention that these patients should return to their families failed to take into account that many may have had very good reason for not wanting to go back to what might ostensibly be called home.

The manipulation of the tax burden from income tax to the poll tax, VAT, local authority rates and national insurance contributions allowed this burden to be shouldered by a less wealthy demographic and increases in economic inequality were compounded by imaginative social security cuts. The 1986 Social Security Act meant a cut of £640 million in housing benefit and a saving of £120 million from a failure to uprate child benefit in line with inflation, a benefit that had already been cut by 21% in real terms.[91] Between 1979 and 1986, the number of people who depended on means-tested benefits rose from 4.37 million to 8.29 million. Relative poverty grew during the 1980s and, in 1985, the sheer depth of the changes prompted the normally benign Archbishop of Canterbury to use his Commission on Inner Cities to attack the government. During this era indirect measures of quality of life such as children's diet and their average height both diminished. Long-term improvements in children's mortality slowed down and more children were ill and homeless.[91]

The 1980s saw a change in the structure of the UK working class. Some were absorbed into an expanded middle class, while many moved into an economic underclass, unskilled and excluded from full citizenship. Thatcher's insistent belief that wealth redistribution was not the responsibility of government meant that this underclass, desperate and isolated, grew from 2 million to 4 million in the seven years following the beginning of Thatcher's premiership. The increase in poverty in the UK far outstripped European neighbours like West Germany, France, Spain, Portugal, Belgium and Denmark, where the trend was for poverty rates to remain constant or decrease during the 1980s. Tony Blair's recent refusal to accept the class boundaries of the UK might come as a surprise to those existing in a very real and excluded underclass.

Stated simply, Thatcherism was profoundly damaging for a great many people in the UK. Policies that encouraged self-aggrandizement and solipsism in commercial and personal life weakened the bonds that tied society together. Escalating unemployment, economic mismanagement and growing social unrest finally prompted her own lieutenants to wield the political axe.

The Caring, Sharing 1990s and Beyond

'8 million people in the UK (1 in 5 of the adult population) owe more than £10,000 through credit cards, overdrafts and loans. One in eight of those with five figure debts say they are quite likely or very likely to declare themselves bankrupt or make legal arrangements to reduce payments. These figures are likely to grow. This survey came from the debt consultancy firm Thomas Charles who found that one in ten of those with large debts struggle every month' *The London Metro, 2006*[96]

In most western countries it has generally been the case that the social democratic or left wing parties have tended to defend the provision of essential public services from those wishing to implement free market fundamentalism. However, the neoliberal acolytes of the 1980s have continued to exert a growing influence over the international political and economic institutions that control our standard of living. Following their landslide victory in the 1997 UK general election, 'New Labour' literally could not wait to embrace monetarism and the two main political parties had formed a new consensus. The recent triumph of market economics and the collapse of any kind of organized and credible socialist political representation have contributed to a profound narrowing of differences between the main parties in both the UK and the US. In the UK, this led to the 'third way' which was actually just the first way carried out by the former purveyors of what I assume could be referred to as the 'second way'. This neglects classic Labour themes of poverty and inequality, a situation supported by the fact that, in the UK and the US, the poor tend not to vote.

Where Thatcher had stolen much of the Labour heartland in the 1980s with her vigorous pursuit of mass home ownership, New Labour returned the favour by embracing what one might hesitantly call a centre-right ideology a decade later. In 1999, the UK Labour government made a big noise about their plans to eradicate child poverty but such an admirable boast was not realized in practice. A real decrease in the percentage of GDP spent on housing between 1997 and 2000 played a significant part in the rise in the numbers of homeless from 44,000 in 1997 to 75,000 in 2002.[75] Continued under-investment in health, education and housing as well as an unparalleled eagerness to embrace part-privatization led to a genuine confusion as to what part of 'Labour' New Labor represented. Indeed the first New Labour term in office saw very little actual change taken to remedy the generation of under investment in the social infrastructure and essential public services. The Thatcherite balance between minimal income tax and increased stealth taxes was continued with gusto by Chancellor of the Exchequer Gordon Brown.[80]

Social Expenditure and Inequality in the 1990s

The late 1990s saw the UK industrial sector continue to contract with the loss of 150,000 jobs between 1997 and 2001. The abandonment of Clause IV and the development of the 'third way' cemented the end of the New Labour project as a centre left concern in the UK. After 1997, the percentage (as a proportion of GDP) of both social expenditure and public expenditure fell, although rising GDP and economic growth meant that a real increase in government expenditure may not have been reflected as a proportional increase. However, the UK remained a low tax country and public services that compare with the best industrialized countries cannot be supported by such a low tax ethos, regardless of how one might manipulate stealth taxes. New Labour has introduced business-speak into the welfare domain and such concepts as creating a welfare system that provides a 'hand up' rather than a 'hand out' have proved popular if somewhat meaningless.

When one thinks of welfare it tends to be in the context of poor and/or unemployed people obtaining money from the tax burden via the government of the day and one tends not to think about the concepts of welfare that benefit the wealthy but the nineties have seen a consistent increase in 'welfare' for the better off. Tony Blair's New Deal used the age-old concept of utilizing the disciplinary properties of welfare by using sanctions to suspend payments if the offer of a job interview was refused. New Labour's New Deal tends to be particularly individualistic in its focus and fails to address the problems associated with affordable childcare and the damage wrought by 'flexible' working practices. For example, childcare credits could not be spent on informal childminders (the likes of which most parents regularly use) but on registered child minders. This is fine except that only 70% of the costs are covered and so it is essentially a credit for those who can afford the remaining 30%. Hence it plays out as a source of welfare for the middle class parent rather than those struggling financially. Meanwhile, the 2002 social fund, the final welfare safety net, has remained below its 1997 level.

The fact that the most egalitarian societies (rather than the wealthiest) have the longest lived citizens has left the US languishing at 19th in the life expectancy of the industrialized countries.[89] Despite, or perhaps because of, a 15% increase in unemployed single parents between 1992 and 1997, 1996 saw the Clinton's administration end 60 years of guaranteed economic assistance to poor parents and their children. Welfare assistance used to function as a reserve army of labor for when times warranted its use.[73] Varying economic cycles meant that such labor would inevitably be necessary when the economic climate took a turn for the better and so a system of welfare kept this store of work at readiness for employment. However, the flexibility of deregulated neoliberal economics has allowed industry to relocate outside of Europe or the US and so this store of labor is simply no longer needed. Welfare has been subject to a campaign of denigration and minimization and those who use welfare assistance have come to be increasingly represented as no more than an economic drain.[73]

Economic growth and employment levels are not always synonymous and managers are now rewarded for downsizing their staff. For instance Thomas Labrecque at Chase Manhattan was recently voted a salary of $9 million as recognition of his progress in eliminating 10,000 jobs.[73] Indeed, the value of shares in AT&T rose significantly when the slashing of 40,000 jobs was announced, an experience that has sadly proved to be the rule rather than the exception. When shareholder profits depend on the reduction of the workforce, we have a perverse situation that will inevitably contribute to poverty and unrest. In such circumstances, falling into the underclass is difficult to view as the choice of the individual but welfare is out of tune with the functions of a modern consumer society and media perceptions of welfare recipients has led to further denigration.[97] While political elites talk about welfare in race-neutral terms, images of black people now dominate US public thinking about welfare and welfare abuse has become increasingly synonymous with welfare. This is discussed in further detail in Chapter 4.

The nineties have seen no reduction in the trend towards greater inequality and economic disparity and by 2002 the richest 1% of the UK owns 23% of the country's wealth (it was 18% in 1986) during a period when the country's wealth has greatly increased.[98] It was reported in 2005 that the number of companies paying seven figure salaries to their directors has passed one thousand and the growing pay of top executives has inevitably contributed to this gap between the wealthy and less wealthy.[99] In 1979, 6% of the national income was received by the top 1% but by 1999 that figure has ballooned to 13%. In the late 1990s the distribution of personal wealth has continued to grow more unequal under the auspices of New Labour and in 2001 Britain was the fourth most unequal country in the European Union.

By 1999, 4.5 million children in the UK were living in poverty and this threefold increase since 1979 meant that, at 32%, the UK has one of the highest rates of child poverty in Europe. To contextualize this, it stands at 13% in Germany and 12% in France and the average in Europe is 20%.[75] Indeed a UNICEF report in 2006 showed that children in the UK were among the worst off in Europe with many living in dysfunctional families and UK children were ranked 21st out of 25 EU countries in child well-being.[100]

From the late 1980s onward inequality and poverty have risen dramatically in the western world. New Labour policies to address this differ very little from those of the previous Conservative administration and social mobility is now lower in the UK than any other advanced country with the exception of our dear old partners in crime, the US.[93] A social exclusion unit was established in 1997 but real policy incentives that might address these issues are simply non-existent. In fact the intentions of the recent New Labour administration have led to regular and considerable rebellion from members of the Labour party in parliament. Forty-seven Labour MPs voted against cuts to lone parents' benefits in 1997, 62 against foundation hospitals and a further 72 voted against university tuition fees in 2004.

It is not only the status of welfare recipients but everyday workers that is changing. A recent study from the Department of Trade and Industry confirmed the government's wishes for the people of the UK to 'work smarter' in order that they experience employee satisfaction.[101] Exactly how working smarter will benefit the populace of a country that already has the longest working hours in Europe (at 43.6 per week compared with 40.3 on the continent[101]) was less clear. The seven years leading up to 2006 has seen a significant rise in the number of employees working more than 48 hours per week (up from 10% in the late 1990s to 26% in 2006) with a whopping one-sixth of the British labour force working at least 60 hours per week. Such figures reflect the continuation of changes in employment procedures and practices that took off in the early 1980s and show no sign of abating. Moreover these employment practices are not necessarily conducive to the physical and mental health of the people who operate within them. Routinely working 12 hours a day increases the risk of becoming ill by 37%[101] but the UK's governing politicians have helpfully manufactured an opt-out from the EU working time regulations that stipulate 48 hours as the maximum working week.

In the US, the poor are quite well hidden from view[86] but inequality has grown in a similar fashion to the UK. The top 20% of the population now owns 84% of the country's wealth and a racial divide is prominent. Whereas the 1999 European American's median income is $44,000, for African Americans it is $28,000 and for Hispanics $31,000. Regarding welfare, The Personal Responsibility and Work Opportunity Reconciliation Act of 1996 repeatedly stated the primary aim of 'eliminating welfare' and addressed President Clinton's pledge to 'end welfare as we know it' when he ran for a second term. To an extent, this has proved true but he did not say that he would replace it, in a great many cases, with poverty.

We are often told that Americans view the welfare state as a European invention[97] that is at odds with a people who like small government and individual self-reliance. Well actually research often proves this argument to be untrue. Year after year, surveys show that most American's do not think that their government is doing enough with regard to health care, child care, education, the elderly and the poor, and most Americans believe that the government should be spending more to fight homelessness and poverty.[97] However what represents the poor and what represents those on welfare is often viewed very differently. In a country already disposed to individualism and self-reliance, Reagan worked to convince many Americans that their falling living standards in the 1980s were a result of expensive and wasteful programmes for the poor. Clinton built on Reagan's manifest welfare cuts by abolishing the Aid to Families with Dependent Children (AFDC) programme and replacing it with the Temporary Assistance for Needy Families (TANF), which gives states a fixed sum to spend on social services for the poor. States can no longer use federal funds for an adult who has been on welfare for more than five years and they can choose to deny welfare to unwed parents under 18 years old or indeed withhold it from women who have additional children while receiving welfare. Welfare sanctions accounted for 20% of the case closures between 1997 and 1999. States with larger minority populations have stricter sanctions and time limits and so racial minorities tend to be disproportionately affected.

The New Face of Privatization: Social Regeneration and Community Planning

Although social exclusion or, as it used to be called, poverty (I never really saw a need for a name change other than to create a concept that is more likely to be judged the responsibility of the excluded. After all no one chooses to be in poverty but some may choose to be 'socially excluded'), and inequality continued to grow through the 1990s, the UK government used what was called the single regeneration budget to fund new developments and improvement schemes to reduce deprivation in the inner cities.[102] Such a process has to be administered by a combination of local people and private bodies who match public funding in order to support local economies. Unfortunately, the needs of local communities and private bodies often clash and have led to a number of projects that could barely be considered to be in the interest of local communities.

It has long been accepted that the loss of a community focus can damage community and local relations with both financial and social implications. For instance local markets serve to draw communities together and community planning is important with regard to maintaining these centers of public interest. However in the UK, distortions in the planning system allow private developers to address their own needs, often at the expense of the people who live in these communities and recourse to appeal against such plans is unique in its paucity. Unlike every other EU country, only private developers (rather than community residents) can effectively appeal against council decisions and so local accountability is removed. This lack of accountability has been behind a series of curious and degrading decisions that have seen local residents suffer at the hands of private developers around the UK.[102]

Local authorities are reticent to deny planning permission to private developers since the costs of going to appeal are prohibitive. Furthermore, the UK is uniquely oriented towards the interests of private developers in that such developers can legitimately provide money or benefits to local authorities as a condition of receiving planning permission. Furthermore, a conflict of interest arises from the Department of the Environment, Transport and Region's dual role as the arbitrars of planning issues in England and their responsibility to promote this sector that they are charged with regulating. This is particularly important since this department grants or withholds permission in controversial and important cases.

The conservative administrations previous to New Labour created the Construction Sponsorship Directorate, an industry lobby that allows easier access to the government with regard to removing regulations that the construction industry found limiting. Such a luminary as John Selwyn Gummer effectively created a lobby to argue for the removal of legislation that he was charged with defending and he took a key role in the development of the Construction Industry Board to actively promote the UK construction industry. Such actions may strike some as a positive contribution to government/business interaction in order to promote industrial success. The more cynical among us may suspect that such relations can lead to private developments that are not necessarily in the best interests of the community as a whole. Indeed such partnerships have led to the current administration's repeated refusal to remove council tax incentives to the owners of more than one home. When communities are no longer able to constructively contribute to the planning process in their area then key decisions about their quality of life are taken by people who will profit from this exclusion of local opinion. Affordable housing will often be sacrificed for the development of luxury homes. New Labour's commitment to this enterprise ethic was emphasized by Richard Caborn when he stated that Britain's regional planning should be business-led. An admirable sentiment when hundreds of thousands of people are homeless and 30,000 elderly die every year due to living in residences unfit for human dwelling.[102]

Stephen Byers – former secretary of state for Trade and Industry, a particular deregulation enthusiast, even by the standards of his New Labour colleagues – was interested in introducing government regulations only where absolutely necessary. Perhaps Byers and his New Labour friends missed the consequences of the previous administration's health and safety executive order to reduce prosecutions of companies who were putting their workers at risk. The subsequent 20% increase in deaths and serious injuries in the workplace, the first time the figure had risen in decades, was obviously nothing to do with the relaxation of such government regulations.

The growth of supermarkets in and around towns is particularly relevant to the short and long-term effects of government regulations on planning. The recent proliferation of superstores and supermarkets has had a number of effects on communities around the country. Figures suggest that the number of superstores in the UK grew from 457 to 1102 between 1986 and 1997. By 1997, 42% of rural parishes no longer contained a shop, a drop unrelated to any reduction in retail food sales. A 1998 government report showed that food shops in towns lost between 13% and 50% of trade with the introduction of a supermarket on the edge of town.[102] Even setting aside the challenge to the community ethic and social cohesion that was previously generated by small shops, employment within a 15 km radius of new superstores is reduced by 5.2% and the local economies of the towns will tend to suffer as money made in small shops previously stayed within the local economies. This money from the local economy is converted into corporate profit, thus contributing to the financial strain experienced by many local residents. The practice of loss leaders, temporary low prices used by supermarkets to drive out local competition, followed by a resumption in normal prices, has been outlawed by recent legislation in Spain, France and Ireland but not in the UK. Moreover, less affluent areas with less mobile resident populations see some stores charge up to 69% more than stores in wealthier parts of the country.[102]

It has been suggested very recently that[103] Tesco, Sainsburys, Asda and Morrisons, which between them control 74% of grocery sales, have built up hundreds of 'land banks' or sites awaiting development. They are now launching a concerted effort to open high street convenience stores and it is feared that such a development will lead to the closure of hundreds of independent stores. The World Trade Organization have recently been lobbied by Wal-Mart with regard to completely removing planning regulations pertaining to size limitations on individual stores, geographical limitations on store locations and numeric limits on the number of stores in a given area. Inverness in Scotland has three Tesco stores that generate 51% of all local spending. This has been blamed for the parts of the city that have now fallen derelict and the associated preponderance of charity shops. Quite simply, few other shops can survive in the vicinity of three Tesco superstores. A recent parliamentary report on the UK high street suggested that retailers such as newsagents, local convenience stores, petrol stations, electrical goods stores, DVD rental and bookshops are particularly unlikely to survive.[103]

So who is currently looking after our planning guidance on the restrictions on out of town supermarkets? Well David Sainsbury, the Sainsbury chain's former chief executive has recently been a minister at the Department of Trade and Industry, which oversees competition policy. Tesco executives inhabit six government task forces including the Department of Trade and Industry's Competitiveness Advisory Group. Such close political links to supermarket retailers is not peculiar to government ministers with such Conservative party luminaries as Francis Maude, the party chairman, proudly operating as a non-executive director of Asda.

This industrial representation of senior figures in the UK political spectrum extends to our hospitals. Trust hospitals can sell land and build supermarkets within their grounds. Not necessarily a problem in and of itself except when we realize that the single largest business interest of members appointed to the boards of 52 out of 57 hospitals that opted out of local health authority control[91] was property development.

Private Finance Initiatives

Between 1997 and 2000, the share of contact hours for home care delivered by independent contractors rose from two-thirds to double that provided by local authorities and in 2004, seven private organizations were contracted to perform 250,000 operations a year over five years in order to cut NHS waiting lists. Indeed, it is in this domain of health and education that the New Labour leaders have pressed home their private sector credentials with the most vigor.

The use of private finance in conjunction with public funds has been a personal crusade for Tony Blair's government. Such schemes allow the government to maintain a tight grip on annual borrowing. They are based on the adage that private management is automatically superior to public management, although this contention is by no means certain. Concerns over the establishment of two-tier systems for health and education have arisen from the development of foundation hospitals and city academies. They have led to significant backbench revolts against the government in the House of Commons, since not all Labour MPs share Tony Blair's zealous enthusiasm about the prospect of multimillionaires running essential public services. One should not assume that a school curriculum designed by a group of conservative, right-wing, enterprise-oriented businessmen is ideal for the broad ranging education of the future electorate. For a £2–3 million donation, the future of the UK can be bought by a group of people who may not always have the best interests of the majority of our citizens at heart.

A considerable conflict of interest arises from the part-privatization of state-owned assets. Such private finance schemes mean that the duty to the public and the duty to shareholders will inevitably collide and it is doubtful that we need to consult Stephen Hawking to work out who is going to come off worse. Anyone with a fiduciary duty to shareholders cannot be said to be working in the best interest of the public and Private Finance Initiative (PFI) schemes will always face this conflict.

Affordable universal healthcare in the UK is under threat as a result of successive government's insistence that private partnerships be shoehorned into the building process for hospital buildings. The way that new hospital development plans impact on the number of beds and doctors is seemingly irrelevant and it has been suggested that the health trusts running the first PFI hospitals will lose a total of 3,700 beds.[102] With what confidence can we say that the private finance NHS hospitals will be administered according to the needs of the patients rather than the needs of the shareholders involved? After all, according to an accountancy firm that advises PFI client companies, most health consortia hope to make significant profits from privately financed hospitals. Indeed, some of the PFI schemes that are cheaper (such as private prisons) achieve this by paying lower wages to staff and providing poorer services.[102]

The criticism that the PFI delivers state assets to private firms is not repudiated by the knowledge that the Confederation of British Industry successfully lobbied for the replacement of the civil servants on the government's private finance panel with a task force of representatives culled from industry. As a result, public accountability vanishes and we are left with a governing task force accountable only to their shareholders.

The 1990s have seen a conglomeration of power in the way that financial, business and political elites have forged closer links, enough so as to warrant suspicion in many cases.[98] The free and seemingly natural movement from being a member of the political elite to the board of privatized companies that benefit from government deregulation initiatives, prepared by legislation from their departments, has no place in a modern democracy and questions the very democratic principles at the heart of the UK and the US governments. Such movement contributes to the cynical attitude of much of the electorate towards politics and the people who inhabit politics. The UK electorate has adopted the attitude that I take to motorcycle riders. Personally I have always believed that anyone who wants to drive a motorbike on the streets should, by definition, not be allowed to do so since they are thrill seekers who represent a constant source of danger (apologies to safe motor cycle riders and flying pigs). Ergo there should be no motorcycle riders on the roads. Likewise the electorate believes that anyone who wants to become a politician is inherently untrustworthy by the very nature of their desire to enter the murky world of politics and such belief leads to the chronically low turn outs that we are currently experiencing for local and national elections. Unfortunately by failing to contribute to the political process, we automatically sanction the monetarist movement of the last 25 years that has led to greater inequality, increased poverty and poorer investment in essential public services.

Chapter 4
Globalization: Definitions and Debates

Having touched upon some of the political and economic changes in the UK and the US over recent years, we now arrive at this nebulous process known as globalization. Indeed many of the structural changes discussed in the last chapter are synonymous with what we have come to know as globalization. The problem is, however, defining globalization. My experience on the topic is that if you read ten different books or articles on globalization you will encounter a number of distinct definitions. However an understanding of this process is crucial if we want to frame the context of the political changes that have happened not only in the west but around the world in recent years. More importantly it will help us to frame the changes that are likely in the coming years; changes that will affect areas as diverse as international trade, employment legislation and work conditions, public services, poverty, welfare, inequality and mental health.

The processes that constitute globalization are primarily represented and shaped not only by western governments, but by international financial institutions like the International Monetary Fund (IMF), the World Trade Organization (WTO) and the World Bank, and by national and international trade organizations and initiatives like the North American Free Trade Association (NAFTA), the Multilateral Agreement on Investment (MAI), the Transatlantic Business Dialogue (TBD) and the European Round Table of Industrialists (ERT). The sometimes ambiguous roles, responsibilities and levels of accountability of these institutions are discussed in order that we try to obtain a clearer understanding of the economic and social changes that we, the world's general public, are experiencing and will continue to experience in the near future.

A glance at the literature on globalization could lead to the conclusion that it is no more than the spread of science and technology through the world and, while some of the advocates of globalization may be content with such a description, it fails to tell the whole story. As a basic description of globalization, it is not erroneous but what such a description fails to do is bestow an appreciation that any such reified process comes to represent more than the sum of such parts. What is important about the spread of science and technology is not the science and technology parts but the 'spread' part. The process used to spread science and technology; the people and organizations responsible for the spreading and what they stand to gain from it; the effects of the spreading process on different countries and different people within countries and the social, political and economic effects of the spreading process are fundamental. Globalization has come to be defined by many as the processes by which such science and technology have been spread. There is no more inherent good or evil in the spread of science and technology than there is in the spreading of a tax burden or the spreading of a corporate brand. How it is spread is all important.

Bill Clinton said that 'Globalization is about more than economics. Our purpose must be to bring together the world around freedom, democracy and peace and to oppose those that would tear it apart'.[104] These were the fundamental twenty-first century challenges that America had to meet. His former cabinet member, Nobel laureate and World Bank mandarin Joseph Stiglitz remonstrates against those who vilify globalization since they often overlook the benefits.[105] He noted that many countries have grown quicker than they would have done otherwise as a result of international trade opening up. While this sounds fine in theory, in practice globalization and the harmonization of international trade has not followed a utopian course allowing the enfranchisement of one and all.

Globalization can and has been represented in a number of ways. We can refer to it through an appreciation of recent changes in science and technology; through the proliferation of western concepts of freedom and democracy in the developing world; and as the creation of closer trade links or as a greater generic international cooperation and cultural appreciation. In a sense all of these definitions have an element of validity. However, what it really comes down to, the fundamental bottom line that underpins a number of other cultural, political and structural changes is the spread of local and global capitalism, in particular, the Anglo-American version of capitalism.

For the sake of simplicity, capitalism can broadly be defined as the private ownership of property, action motivated by profit and free market fundamentalism, and different kinds of capitalism adhere to these three tenets in different ways and to different extents. Globalization has come to represent the movement of the neoliberal economic ideology from the few to the many and it is something that is happening to everyone, whether we are ready for it or not. In the early nineteenth century, capital was static and labour was, to an extent, mobile but today that situation has been reversed and capital is mobile and labour is static so the economic advantage rests on the side of accumulated capital rather than organized labour. As we have seen, companies can move to where labour is cheapest, and multinational and national corporations are able to play one workforce off against another. As such, national governments increasingly administer their economies and electoral responsibilities on the behalf of local and global elites.

What Is 'Bad' Capitalism?

Any discussion of capitalism as a single economic concept is actually bound to failure since it makes little sense to refer to it as a single entity. Different capitalisms have been practised in different areas around the globe with very different political, economic and social outcomes. Anglo-American capitalism, as preached by the US, the UK and New Zealand particularly, has taken the form of a neoliberal ultra-capitalism whose tenets are free market fundamentalism, deregulation, privatization, corporate flexibility, minimal public spending and low taxes. This kind of capitalism re-emerged in the early eighties and was driven by Thatcher and Reagan's immense desire to collapse the social democratic Keynesian consensus that had existed, to a lesser or greater extent, since the Second World War. A series of policy initiatives led to these countries developing a specific type of capitalism that is founded on short-termism, profit as the driving motive for public and private strategy and a focus on the success of the individual at the expense of notions of community or society.

An alternative European capitalism, popular in Switzerland, Germany, the Low Countries, Scandinavia and, to some extent Japan, is based around consensus, collective success and long-term political considerations. The Anglo-American capitalism is social Darwinism writ large, whereas its European variety depends on the relationships between competition and cooperation and is oriented towards trading off losses in short-term efficiency against concepts of increased public good and communitarian representation. The proponents of Anglo-American capitalism have no interest in such a trade off and the general good of the public is not considered to be relevant to the machinations of industry and, to a large and growing extent, government policy, whereas capitalism in Europe is fundamentally opposed to liberalization and individualism. In Germany, the interests of shareholders are represented in combination with stakeholders on company boards and these boards represent employees and local communities.[80] Such a system is based around the development and protection of social cohesion.

The argument is not 'should we have capitalism'? To an extent that is like asking do we want the weather? The argument is which type of capitalism do we want? Globalization is the spread of Anglo-American capitalism into spaces that it did not previously occupy. While prominent authors[105] believe that Chinese, Japanese and US capitalisms are different and cannot be homogenized, this process of attempted homogenization is exactly what is happening under the rubric of globalization, with markedly negative consequences for people the world over. It might seem reasonable at this juncture to ask why the electorate of a country whose economic ethos is focused on public welfare should want to trade it for the endemic social division, growing inequality, insecurity and multiplying ghettos created by US free market fundamentalism? Where is the incentive to move the economic consensus towards a society that has CEOs earning 150 times the average worker when their own economies create far lower inequality ratios?[29,106] Or indeed to move to an economy that has less hospital beds per 10,000 people in the population,[107] a lower life expectancy, lower secondary school enrollment, higher infant mortality and higher carbon dioxide emissions[108] than their own. In France, 54% of GDP is taken up by the public sector and the growth of supermarkets is restricted by controls. Planning issues are controlled by locally elected mayors amid a system that makes sure that small schools and shops are kept open. Why would one want to compromise this? Well generally speaking, most people would not and so the business elite, driven by the short-termism and profit motive of Anglo-American capitalism have moved to paint a picture of mainland Europe as a backward continent, hanging on to the last vestiges of an outmoded economic and political consensus.

In fact there is little to suggest that the opponents of European capitalism are correct per se. European capitalism works if what you want is a form of capital accumulation with consideration towards the effect that such accumulation has on the community as a whole. However many influential supporters of the Anglo-American breed of capitalism have held the US up as a paragon of free market success with the European economic consensus parodied as an entity doomed to inevitable failure. This is the case even though Germany has overtaken the US as the world's largest single exporter, even though relative poverty in the US and UK is considerably higher than their EU competitors (see Table 1) and even though the US is the most economically protectionist country in recent history (western countries committed to neoliberal utopias have long histories of forcing developing countries to eliminate trade barriers whilst maintaining many of their own. The recent US tariffs against cheap Russian uranium and imported steel hardly support their desire for a truly global market for goods).

In this new rivalry, Anglo-American capitalism, egregious to the social welfare of communities and their citizens, will tend to drive out good capitalism[80] with European and Asian social market economies being undercut by economies that can afford to make savings through minimal public investment and few regulations to support the welfare of their workers. Such cuts in investment and deregulation create attractive environments for corporate interests but at the expense of the quality of life, standard of living and social welfare of the people who inhabit them. Indeed it is not impossible to envisage a continuation towards competition for business investment that will lead to an absolute low in the standards of protection that people have recourse to. Indeed rivalry between states in the US has produced just

Table 1 Relative poverty rates of a selection of EU countries and the US and UK. This is the percent of the population that live in three poverty brackets that are represented as a proportion of the middle income of the population (as measured by The 1994 Luxemburg Income Study,[109] a reliable non-profit cooperative research project with a membership of 30 countries on four continents). Data obtained from the Luxemburg Income Study (LIS) Key figures, accessed at http://lisproject.org/keyfigures.htm on 1/8/6

Country	% of population with less than 40% of median income	% of population with less than 50% of median income	% of population with less than 60% of median income
US	10.8	17	23.8
UK	5.8	12.4	21.2
Sweden	3.8	6.5	12.3
Norway	2.9	6.4	12.3
France	3.4	8.0	14.1
Germany	4.7	8.3	13.2
Netherlands	4.6	7.3	12.7

such a socio-political outcome. Rapid population growth in developing countries has eclipsed the influence of organized labour and despite strong and continuous economic growth in western countries in the last 20 years, the number of people excluded from access to employment has continued to grow.

The European and Asian social market economies will struggle to be competitive in the short-term, although not necessarily in the long-term. The success of Anglo-American capitalism will flourish under certain conditions. If you seek short-term profit maximization at the expense of long-term social and industrial success then Anglo-American capitalism will drive out European capitalism because it can undercut it but this is a choice, not an inevitability and the extent to which the business elite can influence the political process and present limited choices as inevitabilities is increasingly important. Success depends on the definition you use. The Japanese practice of employing workers who are economically unproductive in low skilled jobs is not inefficient if your definition of efficiency includes avoiding misery, poverty and social desolation. However, your common or garden neoliberal might view such an arrangement as manifestly inefficient since economically unproductive workers are being needlessly employed, a process that is diverting profits from shareholders to the community. Should pseudo-international institutions like the IMF or international business organizations like the Transatlantic Business Dialogue (discussed in greater detail later in the chapter) lobby for abandonment of Japan's commitment to full employment, a social peace that has been preserved in the country for many years will be profoundly threatened.

Regarding Anglo-American capitalist labour relations, the US no longer possesses a culture of resistance, public or political, to industrial influence and the culture of long hours with few basic benefits or security. The totalitarian nature of the country means that short-hours have come to be considered un-American and a threat to national prosperity. Those who fight this ethos have been represented as national traitors to the cause with the result that 80% of Americans now believe it is impossible to survive on a single income[85]. Business logic suggests it is easier to hire fewer people for longer hours and so an industrial culture has been created where corporate efficiency is promulgated at the expense of the manifest social problems that result from such a culture. These are the kinds of practices that are exported as Anglo-American capitalism takes hold in countries whose national economies seek to keep up with the demands of international commerce. US workers are currently working several weeks more annually than German and Swedish workers[85] but we can expect this disparity to dwindle as European governments are increasingly pressured over the coming years.

In the US and the UK, such untamed capitalism has taken the greatest hold[78] and the devastating effects on the mental health of its populace are discussed in the next chapter. The existence of a functioning, socially cohesive society has been all but destroyed in the US. A longstanding obsession with individualism and individual freedoms, combined with neoliberal capitalism has seen to that. The UK, whilst adopting a similar economic and political revolution over the last 25 years, still has social institutions and cultural traditions that have slowed its transformation into a state governed only by economic and commercial imperatives, but it is catching up.

The current international political consensus reflects the success of the neoliberal politicians and business leaders around the world. The growing weakness of nation states, their government representation, their synonymous movement between positions in the political and business elite and their international political institutions are symbols of their achievement and globalization is the continuing outcome of this success. New technology has allowed global elites to move large sums of money around the world with great alacrity and states that fail to fall into line fail to win international commerce as they cannot provide competitive economic conditions. This is particularly important now that multinational companies account for two-thirds of world trade.

The other side of the equation is that the states that move towards market fundamentalism are no longer able to organize effective social action since their governments become too weak to be able to manufacture meaningful social changes. The interests of shareholders take on increasing importance at the expense of the social, economic and political needs of the electorate. Unlike the citizens of a given state, shareholders are free to move between companies and are not tied to a given space. Recent market fundamentalism is incompatible with basic concepts of democracy because international corporate interests govern the decisions made by national state governments, often at the expense of the quality of life and economic interests of a great majority of its citizens. As the centre of world economic activity moves towards Asia and the Pacific, state activity to improve the life of citizens comes a distant second to the importance of investor confidence and public spending decisions reflect this new focus[106].

Are Free Markets the Problem?

There is a big 'however' though and in the interests of accuracy a fuller appreciation of the way that markets can work should be presented. Market fundamentalism is one way of using markets in a political spectrum but not the only way and indeed absolutism of authority can be as dangerous in the long-term as market fundamentalism. In communist China and the Soviet Union, the centralized economic decision making with a single voice and uniform opinion was undemocratic and led to poor economic consequences over time. Any economy must be sensitive to the consequences of the decisions that are made by a controlling government. It needs to be able to respond to an ever changing environment. If markets are operated with disciplined pluralism, that is, the effective selection of optimal options from a number of possibilities, then they can bring great economic success while at the same time being responsive to the social and communitarian needs of a given population.

Markets themselves are not the problem, rather the way that they have been co-opted within the Anglo-American business model.[110] There is nothing inherent within the organization of markets that guarantees the 'correct' solution, although they do tend towards spontaneous order. A perfectly competitive market has many buyers and sellers but none with sufficient leverage to have a significant influence over price. To achieve such a status, coordination mechanisms produced by government interventions and social institutions are necessary. Corporate power can have legitimacy but we need to ensure that government regulations, competition and pluralism maintain a check on its influence on the social and democratic decision-making process. This, however, is not characteristic of the market fundamentalism of Anglo-American capitalism. The establishment of corporate monopolies, the political lobbying by corporations and the dismantling of effective regulation has led to an exploitation of the democratic process in such a way as to have serious consequences for much of the population who exist outside of the political and financial elite. Keynes said that 'When the allocation of capital is the by-product of the activities of a casino, the job is likely ill done'[110] and the disempowerment of government as an adaptive institution to enforce economic regulation has meant that the needs of the majority will continue to fail to be met.

The American business model is simplistic and naïve. Under this rubric, markets are not tailored towards existing social institutions but are instead geared towards rampant self-interest. This will continue to be the case unless they are properly regulated but such a process of regulation is anathema to the neoliberal ideology. Moreover, there has to be an appreciation that not all services can be effectively provided in competitive markets, whether this be forces of law and order or environmental protection.[110]

The Effects of Globalization

So what have been the effects of globalization or the growing dominance of Anglo-American capitalism? Hobsbawm noted that the era of free market fundamentalism has resulted in a billion people living in dire poverty alongside another billion living in growing splendour and a planet that is becoming smaller and more integrated.[106] About 30% of the world's population is unemployed and the gap between rich and poor is growing at a steady rate. As a result of this integration and relative poverty, disenfranchisement, helplessness and sheer disillusionment are felt by so many. Social cohesion, generally a result of consensus and shared knowledge, has been eroded by this growing disparity in the economic possibilities.

Labour and the communities that have grown around organized labour have become increasingly fractured and the sense of collective identity that has in the past been provided by labour is being eroded as working conditions are subject to corporate flexibility. Financial movement is largely beyond the controls of national governments and many of the past tools of economic policy are not relevant or can no longer be instituted for fear of rejection by business leaders. The resulting growth in poverty that has arisen from this loss of government control has tended to focus on deprivation as hunger as opposed to a focus on the full effects of these economic changes. Rather than hunger alone, which is, of course enormously debilitating, poverty and deprivation mean dreadful housing conditions, a lack of future possibilities or hope for improvement, and weakening social bonds. It means families disintegrating under the pressure of multiple sources of deprivation, greater illiteracy, increased crime and aggression, and physical and mental illness (more of which in the next chapter).

The nature and geography of employment is changing beyond recognition. In the US, there has been a creation of millions of poorly paid jobs in the service sector and a decrease in well-paid jobs in the manufacturing sector.[111] Moreover, the triumphalism of much of the US business community and media tends to ignore this growth in low wage jobs, a growth that has left 30% of the country in paid employment but unable to earn a sufficient amount to lift their family out of poverty[106] and the gradual contraction of welfare has left many poor families worse off than before. Globalization has come to represent the decline of unionization, low wages, flexibility, corporate deregulation, welfare bias, increased poverty and an upwardly distributive bias in national economic policy. Uncertainty in employment is a source of great distress and anxiety for many families and globalization has brought a greater dependency on uncertain jobs. The need for families to rely on two wages is growing and planning a secure future is a luxury not available to many in temporary or agency employment.

Recent crime statistics are one of the many reasons that the infiltration of neoliberal ideology around the globe has not been met with unparalleled enthusiasm. A growing lack of social mobility and opportunities for many mired in poverty and despair, and the associated hopelessness and sense of anomie, have led to an increase in a number of different kinds of crime, crimes which affect the perpetrators and their families as well as the victims.[79] Even in the UK, a bastion of neoliberalist transformation over the last 25 years, the numbers of people incarcerated compares well to the shocking figures in the US. In the UK less than one in a thousand people are incarcerated, whereas the figure is approaching one in a hundred in the US and 28% of the US population now live in privately guarded buildings or housing developments.[80] Not a particularly attractive carrot for the social democratic countries where a third of the population do not feel the need to lock themselves up for their own protection.

Racial and economic disparities in criminal behaviour have led to black people in the US being seven times more likely than white people to be imprisoned, a pattern of behaviour that leads to single parenthood in inner cities and all the financial anxiety and parental struggle that this entails. Many parents in these environments face overwork, stress, difficulties with the financial aspects of child rearing and guilt over being unable to provide in a culture where children are bombarded with images of consumer products. Often the time they can spend with children is insufficient as they struggle to hold down more than one job and many of these inner city children thus lack the kind of guidance necessary to avoid a criminal culture so readily available in the areas with the greatest deprivation.

As welfare is no longer driven by the provision of an available source of labour, rehabilitation has been abandoned as a precept of incarceration. The growing underclass are no longer necessary as producers, welfare is slashed and many people are forced onto the margins of economical existence. Whether they enter the penal system or not, they are discarded from citizenship and the number is growing fast in almost every country.[73] In the UK, the population of prisons has soared in recent years and is up 85% since 1993. Indeed in January 1993, there were 41,561 people in jail in England and Wales. The current population is 77,004.[112] The US incarceration rate at the end of 1994 was four times that of Canada and 14 times that of Japan and the California jail population is now eight times what it was in the early 1970s.[80] There are a number of factors at play regarding the soaring prison population, not least the way crime is defined, but a growing underclass marginalized by 20 years of neoliberal policy features heavily. The economic redundancy of the family, the increase in single parent families struggling to make a living and spend time with their children and the systematic denigration of society and concepts of community mean that prisons are among the few remaining means of social control.

Globalization has so far failed to bring the higher standards of living that many of its acolytes promised and there are no indications that it will do so. The rhetoric of many neoliberal apologists has been organized around such concepts as universal development and this is true as long as by universal you mean those who have vested interests in denigrating the social and economic needs of the majority of the citizens in a given country. Anglo-American global capitalism is focused on the desires and interests of a wealthy elite and the interests of narrow sections of power have become the most important driving force behind the big decisions that are made by governments. The movement of left wing political organizations to the centre right and right of the political spectrum has meant that there is reduced social democratic influence on public power to balance the more destructive results of the marketplace. Moreover the changes described above are not confined to the US and UK. In Germany, one million jobs have been lost in the last five years and many companies are building plants in Eastern Europe, Asia and Latin America. Anglo-American capitalism is gradually eroding all previous forms of economic organization and these problems are going to continue to grow as the power of governments around the world is diminished by the imperatives of a short-term and rapacious capitalism.

The IMF, WTO and the World Bank

In the US, neoliberal ideology and the American business model, which represent the supposed cutting edge of modern economics and a belief in the market as a tool with which to spread political and economic freedom through the world, has provided the impetus for some of the work of economic institutions like the International Monetary Fund and the World Bank in recent years.

To understand the way that these have developed as the bulldogs of neoliberal ideology requires an understanding of their genesis. The IMF and World Bank originated at the end of the Second World War. The IMF, of whom the US has the only veto, was constructed to ensure global economic stability, and the World Bank to help with reconstruction and development following the destruction of the Second World War. Those countries that wished to secure reparation and reconstruction funds from the US had to conform to US requirements on open competition.[111] The institutions were designed with a view to addressing future economic depressions and the IMF would work by placing economic pressure on countries that were not active in maintaining global aggregate demand by allowing their economies to slump.[105] It would also provide loans to countries where necessary. It was established as a public institution from the money of tax payers the world over but reported to the finance ministries and central banks of world governments. Over the years, however, its role has changed beyond all recognition and today the IMF provides funds to countries if they engage in classic neoliberal policies that lead to a contraction in the economy. Indeed a dramatic change occurred in the 1980s as the IMF moved solely from helping countries in crisis to becoming a constant influence in the lives of people from developing countries.

Joseph Stiglitz, a former member of President Clinton's cabinet and former World Bank chief, has provided a scathing account of IMF policies in recent years.[105] He noted that the IMF makes decisions based on a 'curious blend of ideology, bad economics and dogma that sometimes seemed to be thinly veiling special interests'. While these are often unpopular with governments in developing countries, their fear of losing IMF funding leaves them unable to articulate these doubts publicly. Liberalization is the key to IMF thinking, regardless of the consequences it brings and it has been suggested that many of the IMF policies, such as premature capital market liberalization, have actually contributed to global instability. No matter that no country in history (including the US, UK, Germany and Japan) has been able to create sustained economic growth and achieve economic modernity without a considerable degree of insulation to outside influences, usually provided by large-scale government protection and the subsidization of new industries. A need to rush through liberalization has led to sequencing errors that have brought poverty and high unemployment. Countries without adequately strong financial institutions have been opened up for competition too quickly and with devastating results. Of course not everyone loses out in this system of international economic regulation. By obliging countries to adopt anti-inflammatory measures, the US export industry benefits significantly and price liberalization and the growth of low-wage economies usually bring high profits to foreign investors.

Suspicions concerning the reasons for these policies have not been helped by the World Bank and IMF decision-making processes being undertaken out of the public eye, with finance ministers and central bank governors representing the concerns of the business community in their country. Since these often represent companies that wish to see new export markets open up, the resulting IMF policies are not always in the best interests of the developing countries. A growing number of economic thinkers are denigrating the 'one size fits all' model of market fundamentalism,[105,110] since the contractionary policies tend to lead to recessions. Fiscal austerity, privatization and market liberalization are the three pillars of what Stiglitz calls the 'Washington Consensus' and they inform IMF policy. Pushing such policies too far, too fast has resulted in riots in some countries in the Far East, but the inherent short-termism of Anglo-American capitalism means that such policies are inevitable. Furthermore, the huge financial leverage of the IMF means that they are acting from an unparalleled position of strength.

The social costs of these policies can be profound but tend to be viewed as the eggs that need to be cracked in order to make the omelet, even though it has been suggested that the damage caused by the poor timing of such policy implementation actually leads to social and economic problems for many years. Stringent adjustment policies have led to lower wages and less job protection, cutbacks in education and health spending and corruption because they occurred before adequate regulatory frameworks are in place.

So what does globalization mean to the developing countries around the world? Only a very small percentage of the people in the world are 'in the loop' with regard to the globalized society. About 84% of computer users reside in North America and 69% are men with an average income of $59,000. Only 40% of the world's population has daily access to electricity, 80% of the world's population still lacks simple telecommunication access[106] and the gap between the developed and developing countries has been accentuated by the high speed transfer of information. While developed countries embrace new technologies, tradition has come to be the commodity of the disenfranchised; their blessing while the West continues to struggle without all those wonderful gifts of simplicity bestowed upon the noble savage.

The long list of the devastating effects of IMF-sponsored international economic policies has even led the IMF to recently acknowledge that true worldwide development is not progressing evenly, surely a victory for gross understatement.[106] IMF sponsored economic reforms in Indonesia, including cuts in public spending, led to riots against the Chinese (a considerable part of the local business community).[106] Indeed capital account liberalization was considered to be the single greatest factor leading to the East Asian crisis in the late 1990s and the IMF focused on protecting investors (and hence lowering inflation) at the expense of the people of the country that they were supposed to be helping.[80] Pushing interest rates increased non-performing loans and weakened the banks. With banks closing, no recovery was possible due to a lack of available credit for businesses and such a recession has long-term negative economic effects, regardless of what has been suggested by the thinkers in Washington.[105] A fundamental bias towards the business community at the expense of the citizens of these countries betrayed the original ethos of the IMF and betrayed the people of the countries involved.

IMF programmes of restructure also produced outbreaks of famine in Rwanda, Vietnam and Southern Africa, the closing of clinics and schools in former eastern block countries and Africa, not to mention poor working conditions and low pay. The arrival of Wal-Mart and K-Mart in Mexico following NAFTA trade amendments (discussed later) in the mid-1990s has led to stores being driven out of business in their thousands and a $40 billion US bailout to Mexico in order to see off an influx of Mexican immigrants to the US. This poster child for neoliberal reform simply could not be seen to fail.[80]

In the former USSR, IMF sponsored shock therapy has been disastrous for the population and has led to poverty and corruption on an unprecedented scale, with incomes lower and poverty higher than at the end of the 1980s.[105] Without the necessary financial institutions and legal regulations in place to support a capitalist economy, government monopolies gave way to private monopolies and asset stripping with billions of dollars pouring out of the country into suddenly transformed British football clubs, among others. Corruption meant that state assets were sold at incredibly low prices and without an effective tax system. The billions of dollars that the IMF was providing to stabilize the currency supported a corrupt regime.

A fundamental belief in trickle down economics means that growth has often been used to excuse a number of austere and socially disruptive business policies but growth alone simply does not lead to improvements for all citizens. Trickle down economics is not a system of economic action but an excuse for the protection of vested interests.

However, perhaps the most fundamental way in which IMF policies have been flawed in recent years regards the ability of western credit institutions to take advantage of attempts to support the exchange rate.[105] Wall Street regards inflation as the worst evil because it erodes the real value of what is owed to creditors. The IMF, in order to bail out US creditors, provides finance to artificially stabilized exchange rates. Western creditors have little incentive to make sure that whoever they lend their money to can pay if they know that they are going to be bailed out by the IMF. Also, much of the money used by the IMF to stabilize foreign exchange rates goes into the ample pockets of speculators who will take advantage of a given economic crisis. Such events are not unpredictable when we consider that international bankers play such a prominent role in the IMF. Foucault wrote that 'the successes of history belongs to those who are capable of seizing the rules'[113] and, through the IMF and World Bank restructuring programmes, the US have certainly seized the rules. Without accountability and transparency, or a state by state analysis based on economic science rather than a one size fits all free market ideology, without the implementation of strong national governments, many developing countries will continue to suffer at the hands of the US business agenda.

The Trade Organizations

The International Monetary Fund and the World Bank are not the only organizations that have been used to spread US neoliberal policy initiatives at the behest of the US business community. The IMF and the World Bank, with their links to national governments and central banks, are represented by at least a theoretical element of political consensus and international philanthropy. There are also a number of international organizations that have been founded to further influence the political consensus with regards to the needs of the international business community and their actions have led to worrying political changes the world over.

The North American Free Trade Association (NAFTA) is a commercial agreement between the US, Canada and Mexico, designed to encourage free trade and easy capital flow between the countries. It was created in order to open the Mexican economy up to cheaper imports from the US[106] and well-organized lobbying from multinationals meant that the NAFTA came to bear despite domestic political opposition. As a result of the NAFTA, more than a third of Mexican businesses went bankrupt in 1995 and falling wages and disappearing jobs are affecting women disproportionately, since they tend to work in the electronics and apparel industries.[114] Following the implementation of the NAFTA, 28,000 small Mexican firms closed, 334 US firms relocated to Mexico and the Mexican government followed $17.8 billion and $20 billion loans from the IMF and US government with the usual IMF-sponsored initiatives like increased taxes, privatization, increased interest rates and cuts in public spending to reduce inflation.[114] While real wages for Mexican employees have plummeted as a result of the currency devaluation, those linked to the financial sector, particularly investors, have benefited from the changes wrought by the NAFTA.

The Multilateral Agreement on Investment (MAI) was negotiated between members of the Organization for Economic Co-operation and Development (OECD) between 1995 and 1998. The purpose of the MAI was to develop multilateral rules to ensure that international investment was governed in a more systematic way between nation states. The agreement is almost identical to the NAFTA and was proposed and drafted by business leaders. It would have granted corporations the right to sue any bodies whose laws restrict their ability to generate profits.[102] Without being open to appeal, MAI tribunals would be administered by corporate lawyers and would allow corporations to further remove national regulations that exist to protect the indigenous workforce from exploitation from international trade. It would not be an exaggeration to suggest that such an agreement would move towards the replacement of elected democracy with tribunals administered by corporate lawyers.

The MAI, along with the NAFTA, the IMF and the WTO, ensure that government decision-making reflects corporate policy and is minimally affected by the democratic political process both between and within countries. The MAI has been drafted with the intention of creating a single global trading regime that harmonizes US trade regulations with those of other countries around the world. It would internationalize such NAFTA scandals as the Ethyl Corporation suing the Canadian government for banning the sale of MMT, a petrol additive that was considered by many scientists to have dangerous neurotoxic effects.[102] The most effective opposition to the treaty came from the mobilization of a wide range of civil non-governmental organizations and human rights groups. They argued that it threatened the protection of human rights. An important turning point in the campaign against it came when Ralph Nader's Public Citizen obtained a copy of the draft agreement and placed it on the internet. The treaty has yet to be implemented since the French government withdrew from negotiations but the very consideration of such a treaty should be considered an affront to elected democracy with potentially devastating social, industrial and environmental effects.

Further business organizations have operated to ensure profound influence over the democratic process and the effects of these organizations have been more prevalent than many people realize. For instance, the European Round Table of Industrialists (ERI), an influential European Union interest group of forty European industrial leaders, was fundamental to European integration and the development of the Single European Act in 1986. With a view to removing trade restrictions and opening up new markets in central and eastern European countries, the ERI was the main driving force behind the single market and their combined power could be effectively managed to force national governments to subscribe to corporate integration.

Another organization with growing influence is the Transatlantic Business Dialogue (TABD), a group of around 100 chief executives from major corporate players in Europe and the US. It was established in the mid-nineties in order to identify trade barriers and opportunities where liberalization could be effected by governments. The TABD identifies these opportunities and submits their proposals to governments[102] with the full expectation of satisfactory action. The TABD has already proved to be profoundly important in influencing the US government to force NAFTA terms on African countries under pain of losing US aid and/or trade and investment.

Such organizations like the MAI, the ERT and the TABD have been created to oversee the implementation of market forces into the political institutions that currently govern our day to day existence and the effects of this continued implementation will prove to be increasingly deleterious to the citizens who labour under their terms. In the 1999 round of trade talks in Seattle, the US and the UK were the driving forces behind implementing further privatization within the EU and this should come as little surprise. We are currently witnessing what might euphemistically be called a battle between the neoliberal free marketers and the less neoliberal free marketers for the heart of Europe and corporate interests around the world have been mobilized to drive through a series of changes that makes Anglo-American capitalism a reality the world over. Whether it is through the NAFTA, the IMF or World Bank, or through the organizations above, the processes of government that protect the rights and quality of life of citizens around the world are being compromised by the institution of changes that meet the needs of a small elite, driven by maximizing shareholder profits via the exploitation of new markets. The effects of such changes will be discussed in greater detail in the next chapter with specific reference to the mental health of the populace.

When being introduced to information on the different organizations, trade groups and treaties that create the agenda under which most of us live, it is easy to be skeptical about the alarmist tendencies of those who introduce such information. This information on these bodies has not been provided to provoke alarm or to scare but simply to tell the story of what is happening in modern political circles and the ways that the political process is being influenced by small groups of powerful people.

Globalization and Consumer Culture in the Last 30 Years

The movement in the west towards the accumulation of capital has meant that every aspect of modern culture that can be commodified will be commodified, almost irrespective of the way that this impacts on the quality of life of the people who live in these societies.[106] Almost all parts of modern society, from art to human body parts, from childhood to mental distress to sports teams, have gradually come under the control of market logic and usually with negative consequences for the great majority of people who do not constitute the major shareholders of the corporations involved. Having inherent cultural value as an artifact itself becomes less relevant than how a given artifact can be exploited for financial gain. The problem with this approach is that it has had a tendency to incorporate people as well as consumer products. This has contributed to a number of the problems that strike at the very heart of modern living.

In the nineteenth century, the US addressed the paradox of living with the possibility of enormous material profits and the social problems inherently linked to unregulated capitalism. They emphasized the principal of equal opportunity with regards to wealth and prosperity. Great prosperity was open to all and rewards would automatically be furnished upon those who had the right work ethic. This principal allowed the dispositional apportioning of idleness upon the indolent and poverty-struck whilst pedaling the concept of the American Dream, that anyone could be anything they wanted with the right approach. Individualism, an already prominent ideology in the US, took off with gusto during the end of this century with, as mentioned in Chapter two, pseudo-scientific practitioners like the Mesmerist Phineas Quimby and Mary Baker Eddy of the New Thought Practitioners arguing the corner for the enfranchisement of the self as a primary motivation.[54] Indeed, the parallel growth of advertizing and psychotherapy was no coincidence as both sought to find space as panaceas for a new consumer society where the service sector was finding new ways to create needs in the population.

A stagnating economy is a poor consumer economy, since consumers are not providing the necessary demand for trade. We saw the generation of what Cushman[54] calls the 'empty self', the idea of systematically convincing the general population that there are consumer products that they need to own. Not that they might want to own or might like to own but that they needed to own whether for personal and social success, occupational well-being, physical health or wealth acquisition. Advertizing grew to provide the rationale for these needs and worked to generate this feeling of the empty self, a self that is somehow missing the products that will make it better, happy, healthy or whole. Psychotherapy grew in conjunction with this ethos. The mental healing industry was perfectly placed to address the needs of these empty selves so successfully promoted by consumer advertizing. Both industries utilized the practice of collecting information about people's lives, their needs and their wants, and sold their products as the solution to people's lifestyle problems. This growing role of the mental health industry is covered in detail in Chapter six.

The development of the modern consumer society received an enormous boost between the two world wars. The use of hire purchase multiplied twenty times, allowing many families to bring household goods and consumables to their homes that were previously out of reach.[115] Banks developed personal credit to allow people to afford the non-essential products and services that would quickly come to be obsolete. Credit sales grew and by 1966 they accounted for 10% of all consumer expenditure. The percentage of after-tax income that Americans saved was less than 2% in 1986, a drop from 26% from the end of the Second World War.[54]

While consumerism took off unreservedly, it did so initially around familiar class and gender divides. In the UK, bargain basements in department stores separated the wealthier patrons from the 'riff-raff' who did not have to enter the main part of the store.[115] Mass consumerism had failed to be sufficiently refined so as to overcome typical class politics. However this would soon change as the working classes were able to substantially increase their credit following the Second World War. Although the division of the classes may not have been quite so sharply defined by their ability to consume, they were still separated by what they could consume. Modern consumption has always been characterized by products initially being available to the wealthy and then moving through the wealth scale until they are eventually afforded by the majority. Sex differences in consumerist behaviour tended such that men took a disproportionate interest in forms of consumption on which status depended, whereas women were left to balance the books, often only buying items with their husband's approval. Advertizing reflected and drove such distinctions during the post-war period.

In the US, GNP increased by 114% between 1940 and 1960, and consumer choice was presented as one of the most patriotic of American values. Consumer choice represented freedom, whether it was freedom to buy or not to buy, this personal and consumer freedom represented what it meant to be an American. Western advertizing has always been able to represent itself in liberationist terms; slogans address the need to fill feelings of internal emptiness that have usually been perpetuated by the same advertizers. Solidity and wholesomeness would be presented as the end-product that could only be achieved by owning a particular brand of make-up, washing machine or low calorie soft drink. Americans could contrast their own consumer culture with that of their cold-war adversaries and it took little time for such a totalitarian democracy to elevate consuming itself an act of patriotism. Furthermore, the youth-driven retail economy started in the late 1950s and early 1960s as advertizers worked to persuade teenagers of the need for certain clothes, music and magazines in order for them to pursue distinctiveness, their own personal brand. This led to young people turning to shopping as a leisure activity, a hobby rather than a function or chore.[115] Such an activity allowed them to separate their world from the staid, old fashioned world of the adults around them and youth consumption was suddenly given wheels. It was used as a tool to challenge the post-war adult society and it continued to grow as real consumer expenditure increased by 60% between 1951 and 1981. Indeed, consumer installment loans grew to 20% of personal income in 1987, a figure that had previously stood at 5% in 1949. Although it was the generation of baby boomers who first used mass consumerism as a tool to draw boundaries between their culture and the culture of their parents, it was their children that really took the baton and ran with it in the explosion of consumerism that was the 1980s.

The growth of television and advertizing in the 1970s and 1980s meant that advertizing retained an influence like never before. More and more people were exposed to the magical benefits that consumer products could bring to their families. The manifest emptiness, social and economic inequality and disablement that so many would come to experience could be ameliorated by the new electric egg whisk or the new video recorder on the market. Social value was coming to be defined by purchasing power and material possessions and television advertizing continued to drive this need for the new, the modern, the exciting and the fashionable. Charles Kettering, general director of General Motors noted that 'business needs a dissatisfied consumer, its mission is the organized creation of dissatisfaction'[85] and while such a synopsis may appear extreme, it was not wholly wide of the mark. A modern consumer society demands a lack of satisfaction and sense of restlessness.

The 1980s and the Success Ideology

So are the effects of modern consumerism really such a bad thing? On the one hand it provides people with the products and services that they want and that most of them can afford and such unalloyed spending supports the local and national economy. After all, these are products that people want.

While this may be true, there are a number of drawbacks to this kind of western ultra-consumerism that should temper our enthusiasm. One might be forgiven for thinking that consumerism is an ahistorical part of human nature, a gene-driven phenomenon that sends us salivating into the nearest high street store. This is not, however, the case.

For the baby boomers, affluence and consumer advertizing led to a level of lifestyle expectations that had not been previously realized. The 'shop till you drop' syndrome became particularly prevalent in the 1980s and not since the 1920s had the US been so tolerant of unrestrained materialism and greed.[85] People had gone from desiring a way of life to expecting it and failure to experience these consumer necessities led to a subjective feeling of consumer and personal disenfranchisement like never before. As the 1980s wore on, consumer remedies were presented as the solution to almost all lifestyle problems, many of which were increasing as the policies of Reagan and Thatcher brought new levels of inequality, poverty, occupational unpredictability and personal and political isolation. The self-improvement industry via diet, cosmetics and electronic equipment grew to be great providers of fulfillment and growth, although this 'cure by consumption'[54] meant that many of those living in poverty were disadvantaged not only by their existing in a state of grim despair but by their inability to access the cure, beamed into their front rooms every day on television. Overspending, overextended credit and economic anxiety was promulgated by advertizing aimed towards both those with a considerable discretionary income and those without.[89] It was not unusual for people to use consumption as a way of coping with feelings of unhappiness and distress, as a way of sating emotional needs. The feeling of being constantly dissatisfied, devalued, isolated and discontented came to dominate many people's lives.

The growth of the middle classes allowed for the creation of a large group of potential buyers whose increased productivity has been used to raise incomes to engage in further consumption rather than supplement a reduction in working hours.[85] For the 20 years following the early 1970's, the amount of time Americans spent at their jobs rose steadily with inevitable results. Parents devoted less time to their children, experienced increased stress and often struggled to maintain the balance of work and family. Schor characterizes many Americans as having been caught up in the cycle of 'work and spend' with people working longer hours in the US than in any other country.[116]

Such work and spend habits continue to the present day. People increasingly look to consumption to provide satisfaction, since their leisure time is gradually diminishing. The poor are simply seen to be not as good at consuming as the wealthy; they are flawed consumers and it is not unreasonable to suggest that this may contribute to their feeling degraded or left behind, isolated from a society that engages in practices from which they themselves are excluded. Many of the poverty-stricken and poor have a great deal of free time and crime has been characterized as a way to engage in the sensation-driven consumer ethos when you are unable to actually consume. Boredom is ameliorated by activities that generate the sensations of consumerism.[73]

While economic growth is celebrated, many of the problems inherent in poverty are exacerbated if economic growth is accompanied by greater inequality; where the benefits of such growth are disproportionately spread among the wealthy, as is the case at present in the UK and the US. Glaring inferiority is heightened by the visible displays of consumption of the wealthier sections of society. Many people find this bearable but it becomes less so if their children are suffering, since the results of such consumer inequality tend to be most savage in the play-ground. More US children than anywhere else believe that their social status is defined by brands and clothes and hence show more brand affinity than children anywhere else in the world.[85] Children are bombarded with consumer messages that show that products and services equate to happiness and satisfaction. Oddly enough some of these children are sent to behaviour modification camps in the hopes that harsh, consumption-free environments will cure them of problems that have arisen from the learning of the consumer codes. Parental guilt has become all too common as children are exposed to mass consumer advertizing on television and the relative affluence of some classmates. If happiness and contentedness are represented by the purchase of certain objects, and these objects are out of their reach, then the inability to maintain certain consumer lifestyles becomes the inability to maintain happy lives.

Consumerism in Schools, the Media and Advertizing: Anglo-American Capitalism for a New Generation

There was enormous media expansion in the 1980s and this meant that advertizing in Europe doubled between 1980 and 1987, an expansion that continued well into the 1990s. Indeed, global advertizing will increase at a greater rate than GDP growth for the foreseeable future as the rest of the world elevates its advertizing potential to that of US proportions.[117] The limited enforcement of antitrust statutes and regulations in the US have been reduced to the point of irrelevance. From abroad, the ability of nation states to control their advertizing content has reduced with the growth of satellite and cable television. For instance the Geneva-based court of the European Free Trade Association ruled that Norway could not prohibit advertizing to children, as was previously their policy, on satellite broadcasts from outside of the country. Similarly, in 1996, the European Court of Justice ensured that Sweden could not ban advertizing to children if the broadcasts originated outside of Sweden.[117]

The way that advertizing influences children has changed in the last twenty years and the UK and the US have led the world in initiatives that allow more children to be exposed to corporate influence in education and advertizing (and at an earlier age) than ever before. The European Round Table (ERT) see education as a prime market opportunity and one that should be treated as such.[102] Industrialists and entrepreneurs have come to view education as far too valuable to be placed in the hands of such unworthy denizens as public servants who continually impede the path of commercial progress. As such, ERT lobbying has led to the UK's Education Action Zones where corporations give schools sums of money that are matched by government contributions.

Such firms as British Aerospace have become involved in Plymouth, Hull and Teesside[102] and Lambeth's Education Action Zone aims to 'increase understanding and experience of employer culture'. It is not unreasonable for some parents to question whether their children will come to identify with the companies in the sense that they will accept the morality of the market. For those who do harbor these fears, the prediction that 200 state schools will be managed by private companies in the UK in the very near future is a frightening prospect.[102] Together with part-private funding of city academies, Tony Blair's personal pet project, the privatization of UK education is moving forward apace.

In the US, there has been an explosion of school-based marketing since 1997 and the influence of Channel One, the daily news and advertizing channel, has increased.[116] About 40% of US secondary schools (and usually the poorest) have signed deals with Channel One communications. In return for its programmes being shown to 80% of pupils nearly every day, televisions, VCRs and satellite dishes are provided to the schools. It is thought that 8 million students view these programmes, an audience second only to the Superbowl.[116] What is important about Channel One is not the news coverage that children are exposed to but that the news is delivered with two minutes of commercials on sets with volumes that are not adjustable. The commercials have represented such activities as military recruitment and have been used to promote tobacco brand names. Students exposed to Channel One commercials are more likely to agree, as a result of their being shown in the classroom, that the products advertized are good for them. It is not necessarily surprising that children should make such a link if they are exposed to advertizing in an austere environment normally reserved for learning. The practice of giving teachers from non-Channel One schools kickbacks if they can bring their schools 'on board' has been particularly effective in the recruitment process.[116]

Channel One is not the only provider of such services. ZapMe! has provided computers to schools in return for exposing children to adverts online for a given amount of time every day.

A relatively new practice called 'pouring rights' is characterized by school districts holding exclusive contracts with soft drink companies. This was debuted in 1997 and the questionable educational value of baking 'coke cakes' and devising marketing plans for Coke discount cards is a concern for some parents. Advertizing has also moved into other aspects of the childhood experience with sponsorship of athletic teams, stadia, gymnasia and sports activities common-place. Companies like Youth Marketing International claim that 92% of teachers use its programmes, consisting of essential educational learnings like how to design a McDonald's restaurant.[116] Since such projects are being disproportion-ately taken up in poor schools, it is not unreasonable to suggest that those children who are least likely to be able to afford consumer products are those who are most exposed to their advertizing, an advertizing process that has again been given added gravitas by their being placed in a school context. When the attempts of Maryland's legislatures to ban adverts and soft drink contracts in public schools are defeated by lobbying from Channel One and the soft drinks industry,[116] we can begin to understand the insidious nature of how initiatives like the MAI could function in everyday society were they to be ratified globally. The importance of government regulation to keep the area of school and public education free from the cynical effects of advertizing is fundamental but such regulation is constantly under attack in the UK and the US. The end product of such deregulation in schools is highlighted by the fact that, despite 78% of US parents being opposed to or strongly opposed to brand advertizing being shown in schools,[116] the practice continues. The arguments of companies who suggest that parents have an element of control over this process do not stand up when one considers that they are exposed to the advertizing when not under supervision by their parents.

This growing corporate influence in the lives of US children began, not surprisingly, with the Reagan administration's purely selfless desire to increase corporate activity in public schools. Such an increase in commercialization has resulted from the under-funding of schools in both the UK and the US where it is thought that the average teacher spends $521 of their own money on classroom materials.[116]

A Child's Response to Advertizing

So how does regular exposure to advertizing influence children, other than a sense of frustration at being bombarded with adverts about products that many are unable to buy? Well first let us look at the statistics. It is thought that in the US, the average 8 to 13-year-old child is watching 3.5 hours of television everyday although this figure is considerably higher for black and hispanic children. There has been a jump in advertizing spent on children from $100 million to $15 billion in the US since 1983 and the purchasing power of children has also risen rapidly.[116] With regard to television, it is thought that 44% of children from 4th to 8th grades report daydreaming 'a lot' about being rich and children who watch more television have a greater bias in their perception of how wealthy American people are, since they are exposed to a disproportionate number of wealthy people on television.[116] Perhaps not surprisingly, consumer desires are greater in the children who watch more television, a practice not always under parental control as having both parents at work is quickly becoming established as the norm.

Such consumer advertizing and exposure is disproportionately influencing poorer children and black and hispanic children. These children are exposed to ideas of cool that are sold as 'having something that others do not have' and wealth and the aspiration for material products is often conveyed as obligatory. The reality is that children whose parents are unable to keep up with their child's consumer demands will suffer amongst their peers in a way that adults never would. Greater inequality twinned with greater exposure to commercials will continue to represent a growing number of children as unsuccessful consumers, a crime among their peers.

The greater exposure of children to consumer society both inside and outside the school environment can also have negative consequences for the health and well-being of the child. A survey of 300 children aged between 10 and 13 years in Boston, Massachusetts, showed that 63% of them wanted to make a lot of money when they grow up, a trait that appears to be higher for children from relatively poorer neighbourhoods. The research showed that children who were more involved in consumer culture were more depressed, more anxious, had lower self-esteem and greater psychosomatic complaints and the nature of the analysis showed that the negative psychosocial consequences were caused by consumer involvement rather than the other way around.[116] It was also shown that those who were more consumer-oriented tended to socialize less with peers, parents and siblings. Put simply, the poorer you are, the more likely you are to engage in consumer culture and suffer the negative psychological and social effects associated with such engagement.

The corporate influence over childhood has grown profoundly in recent years with growing influence and market power for megacorporations like Viacom, Disney and AOL Time Warner. Such corporate monopolies have meant less value for consumers and less influence over the ethical standards that our children are exposed to as they grow up. For instance, the corporate finance provided to the major two political parties in the US (Philip Morris gave $9m to both parties between 1995 and 2002, AOL Time Warner gave $4m, Disney $3.6 m, etc.)[116] will allow corporations greater input to the debate on children and advertizing. As discussed above, the effects of this have not always been positive.

Finally, there is a conservative irony at the heart of the way that children engage with consumer culture. This irony is created by the clash of values of old conservatism and new conservatism. The commodification of 'street' has been successful. It is edgy and supports connotations of violence and civil unrest, aspects that pull the child further from the parent and closer to the product. Parents and teachers are portrayed as idiots and creeps and authority comes to exist only with the corporate sponsor. While many conservatives have hijacked this occurrence in order to frame their traditional values, they have failed to recognize that it is their free-marketeering, anti-regulation culture of corporatism that has led to this anti-adult sentiment. Giving children freedom and intellectual and social liberty is not egregious per se. It is, however, dangerous when their agenda is dominated by corporate imperatives. The adult as gatekeeper model is no longer viable.

Globalization and the Media

Much of the media play a crucial role in controlling the political and economic agenda in Western countries and while the UK and the US are quite rightly lauded for their free press, the extent to which it is completely free is debatable. As highlighted by Rupert Murdoch's partial consolidation of the British print press discussed in the previous chapter, advantageous reciprocal relationships between politicians, governments and the media elite are age-old and will continue ad infinitum. It could be argued that such relationships have played an especially important role in many media representations of the political and economic changes in the US and UK in the last 20 years. It is not uncommon for network news bureau chiefs to come directly from the world of politics without backgrounds in journalism and, indeed, for journalists to have achieved their positions through their political rather than journalistic backgrounds.[98]

Having control of media outlets means having tremendous influence on modern society and the democratic process. Private systems of media control tend to be politically conservative and represent a narrow band of interests, usually servicing a small elite who align media output with corporate interests. By the 1970s, the global media system was dominated by mostly US trans-national corporations (TNCs) and was largely profit-driven. The realities of neoliberal policy crept into 1980s national broadcasting and telecommunication at the expense of public ownership and traditional regulations. Indeed, the commercialization of national television systems has been essential to achieving greater control of the consumer process.

The global media system today is characterized by the domination of three or four TNCs.[117] Much of the information that arrives from the media comes from a small number of corporations such as News Corporation, Disney/Cap Cities, TimeWarner and Viacom and associated press agencies like CNN, BBC and Reuters. Public service standards and citizen participation in public affairs, as well as our understanding of public issues, have drastically reduced as a result of the centralization of power in the modern global media system. We now have a population less informed and less able to make political choices as state-controlled broadcasting services continue to experience enormous pressure from the centripetal media behemoth that is bestriding the globe. Perhaps not surprisingly, the result of this tendency to consolidate power in the media is the creation of content that supports the political and economic consensus that creates it.

The media is far from immune to the interests of advertizers and advertizers are interested in paying for some things but not others. Having their adverts in the middle of a discussion that encourages the questioning of corporate power or the influence of advertizing in modern media and politics is not top of their list and so media focus and output will always be prone to influence from more than just current affairs. The perspective used to present the news is all-important and since the late 1980s the UK and the US press has tended to focus on the process of modern politics at the expense of focusing on the actual substance of the values presented.

In recent years, the IMF has worked, with limited success, to open up foreign media markets to worldwide competitors (the US) such that competition can be introduced that will have the effect of allowing greater US corporate control of media output around the world. The phenomena of globalization inherently include the creation of a 'soft media' driven by convenient alliances. Journalism will very rarely question, or question adequately, the process of globalization and its corollary of global justice. Virtual Images and information circulate relentlessly in order to create a media production of news as entertainment as opposed to news as information. Some might argue that this has always been the case. Indeed, the 1930s use of the media to turn the public against industrial action in the US is a case in point.[118] I simply contend that the recent relationships between the media, political and corporate elite have magnified the process.

The Media, Globalization and Representations of Poverty

One of the areas where the media have been fundamentally complicit in following a conservative agenda is representations of wealth and income disparities. These rarely appear in a mainstream media,[86] which is focused on presenting a picture of the world that tends to defend rather than challenge the social, economic and political consensus. Indeed, the way that mass media has been used to frame the causes of poverty is particularly instructive. In recent years, the episodic framing of poverty has been significantly greater than the societal framing of poverty.[119] That is, the US public have been party to more stories about how poverty is centred around individuals and their dispositional flaws rather than treating poverty on the level of social factors. When it is framed in more thematic terms people are more likely to assign responsibility to social phenomena like failed government programmes and initiatives, the political climate and economic conditions. However, if episodic framing is used then people will tend to blame the poor themselves. As such, the media presentation of such a topic as inequality and poverty is absolutely crucial and many years of individualistic poverty images in the media have borne fruit.

Recent research with students shows that white respondents are more likely to make individualistic rather than structural attributions for poverty, although this is not the case for black respondents who, along with Latinos, rate both types of account as important.[120] Furthermore, the causal nature of the poverty experienced by the white poor has tended to be represented predominantly as societal, whereas the opposite has been true of representations of the black poor. Indeed, being a black single mother has been particularly represented in terms of individual personal responsibility.[86] It has been suggested that many white Americans view black people as lacking the American work ethic,[97] and view them as the principal exponents of welfare abuse, this insidious force that, according to Reagan, was holding America back. The perception of welfare abuse in the US is widespread and tends to be associated with lazy blacks and this perception of black indolence is the most powerful predictor of the opposition to welfare shown by so many white Americans.[97]

Today it is undoubtedly dangerous for political and media elites to directly represent welfare in anything other than race-neutral terms but indirect media representations tell a different story. Before the 1960s, US media images of the poor had tended to focus on Appalachian farmers but the migration of black people from the south to the cities, the civil rights movement and consequent battle for economic parity focused public attention on black poverty. An analysis of the media focus from 1967–1992 is revealing. Prominent US publications like Newsweek and Time magazine represented black people in 53% of their images of poverty when the proportion of black poor during the time was actually 29%.[97] Further analysis showed that stories critical of welfare abuse tended to contain pictures of black people, whereas pictures of whites tended to accompany stories on unemployment policy. Generally, there was a lack of black faces attached to any stories that were sympathetic to the poor and since the magazines analysed had a combined circulation in the region of 10 million, one can appreciate the public perceptions that such a bias could create. This bias was evident not only in the written press but in the television news and, since people are more likely to remember what they see on televised news as opposed to what they hear,[97] this image bias has been profoundly influential.

Sections of society with less political and financial power such as the poor, ethnic minorities and women are less likely to have their interests reflected by mainstream media, especially when those interests contradict the interests of the media owners. As such, the difficulties that they face will often be shown to be devalued or misrepresented in the interests of maintaining a given status quo. Media figures benefiting from close political connections to the growing right wing and centre-right neoliberal consensus, whose interests are served by government deregulation of the media industry and occupational flexibility, low tax and lower public spending, will not be leading the bandwagon for changes in the way that current institutional practices perpetuate social and economic inequality.

The media present the interests of the wealthy as the general concerns of the people of the country because they are the interests of the people who own and direct the media.[121] Hence our daily reminder of how the financial indexes are performing when a minute proportion of the population actually know or care about what this represents. Structural economic concerns are downplayed and shared interclass concerns like crime are emphasized in order that the politically and economically disenfranchised are exposed to these 'universal' concerns. The damaging effects of Anglo-American capitalism/globalization and the fact that in 1999 the wealthiest 1% of the population received as much income after tax as the poorest 38% combined will not be coming to a screen nearby soon. Together with the media, popular entertainment shows like Jerry Springer and Ricki Lake present a picture of a working class zoo culture where negative images of poor people become cemented in the public domain.

Welfare recipients become stereotyped as immoral and are subject to general disgust; mostly black scroungers taking the easy option. The fact that the largest group on welfare in the US is poor children is irrelevant since it is single mothers, the paragons of modern immorality and neglect, who fit the picture more conveniently and hence become the focus of attention. If people are not exposed to poverty or to a balanced discussion that covers such structural elements as affordable housing, the preponderance of low paid, temporary jobs and childcare problems, then an understanding of the economic conditions of a great many people in the country will be inaccurate.

This section is not included to build an argument that supports the view of the media as Machiavellian monsters, savaging the poor and wheeling out lies to protect their own growing interests. Rather that the beliefs and perspectives of the decision makers in the media are over-represented and with dangerous effects. This has resulted in bias with regard to representations of welfare, poverty and race, crucial determinants to the development of an informed electorate. What we understand as globalization is a way of life and the neoliberal movers and shakers of the last 30 years in the US and the UK have not had to stretch themselves to convince the media to get on message.

Globalization and Alienation

Margaret Thatcher did not believe that it was the duty of the government to create a sense of community. Rather it was their responsibility to release the energies of individuals whose enterprise and independence had been imprisoned by the state and by society[92] and recent changes in the community ethos of the UK and the US would doubtless have pleased her. Social capital, the strength of social networks and associated norms of reciprocity, has diminished markedly over the last 30 years[122] and such social factors as family cohesiveness, availability of local help and the positive attitudes of other people in the community have fallen in a number of different domains.[47] These changes in civic engagement have been attributed to a number of factors and have been suggested as symptoms of a terminal decline in modern society.

It should be noted however that the history of civic engagement in the US and the UK tends to be a story of ups and downs rather than one long, slow decline. That said, there is little doubt that over the last 30 years, we have been separated from what we previously understood as our communities. After the sense of collective solidarity following World War II, we are now experiencing chronic lows in social capital. In the 1970s, 66% of all Americans attended club meetings, whereas this figure had inverted to 66% who never attended club meetings by the 1990s. Parents are less involved in their children's education than before and the fraction of employees belonging to trade unions dropped by more than 35% in the US between 1980 and 1997. We now feel more rushed than we ever did previously and our political participation has dropped from 63% at the 1962 US presidential election to 49% in 1996 (and this is not just due to a drop in the quality of the candidates, although this may have played a part). Social capital has been replaced with financial capital as more and more people want to engage in 'chequebook' civic engagement rather than attending any grassroots citizen networks.

Our everyday engagement in our communities, from the standpoint of being involved in public affairs, has dropped drastically. Between 1973 and 1994, the number of US citizens who attended one public meeting on school or town issues in the previous 12 months dropped by a remarkable 40% and formal volunteering, community work, informal helping, charitable donations and even giving blood have all fallen considerably during this period.[122] Americans who are more active in community affairs are more likely to give blood but since this kind of citizenry is dying out, so too are associated acts of benevolence and altruism. With regard to religion, there has been a growth in evangelical religious participation at the expense of less individually based forms of worships and so a diminution in the social betterment programmes associated with more traditional forms of religious participation. A long slump in church membership and the associated civic responsibility has contributed to this civic disengagement in recent years.

We are socializing less and less every year while the proportion of adults who live alone has doubled between 1977 and 1998.[122] The number of times that Americans spend evenings with people in their neighbourhood has fallen by a third in the same time period and participation in youth sports, membership of formal and informal social networks and time spent eating together as a family have all dropped significantly over this period.

Enterprise culture and the rhetoric of individualism have spread ferociously with the result that popular culture has legitimized the perception of the self as little more than a consumer. Choice, freedom and individualism grew to be the by-words of an era where rights overshadowed responsibilities, the very responsibilities that a communitarian ethos needs to survive. The growth in the number of televisions owned, the number of channels available and the form, content and sheer saturation of advertizing that people were exposed to provided an effective medium for this growth in enterprise culture. Entertainment through television became increasingly individualized and by 1995 television entertainment (and the associated exposure to advertizing) had grown to absorb almost 40% of the average American's free time.[122] More than 30% of the television watching of children between the ages of 8 and 18 is undertaken alone and such viewing tends to be disproportionately correlated with poverty and lower education.

An increasing emphasis on individualism goes hand in hand with free market economics and neoliberal ideology and the already-strained community bonds that exist within the US and the UK are experiencing further damage with the growing poverty, financial inequality, homelessness and hunger experienced by many on a day to day basis.[89] The UK post-war expansion in housing led to the disruption of existing communities as families with young children were placed in isolated blocks of flats.[123] Indeed, limited social networks and family disintegration in areas of widespread poverty have been known for many years and this growth in poverty and inequality has contributed to the isolation.[124] In a UNICEF report, Sylvia Anne Hewlett characterized the Anglo-American political model as a 'war against children and families'.[79] Previously, the whole family and community were involved with child-rearing, with standards of justice and opportunity promoted by community institutions like schools, churches, day care centers and the extended family. However, as society has become less anchored in the more traditional structures like family and community, it has also become less humane and generally less tolerant.

This does not mean that we must automatically hark back to a better time like some nostalgic granddad with an enormous pair of rose-tinted spectacles. Otherwise, we might fall into the Thatcherite trap of using the family as a convenient solution to structural problems; justifying care in community by sending the mentally ill back into the throng of their dearly beloved despite their often not being welcome or being petrified at the thought of returning to the source of their distress. The family and, indeed, community are not some all-powerful panacea that solves the ills that plague society. However, a loss of focus on the plight of others goes hand in hand with individualism and enterprise culture.

Work and Alienation

The changes in social capital that I have discussed in the different domains above are also reflected in the employment sector with the unionized portion of the workforce reducing in recent years. The un-unionized manufacturing and public sector jobs that sustained an earlier generation have largely vanished.[125] The new workforce of female and white collar, knowledge-based work, view collective bargaining as less relevant and the cult of the individual has spread to the work environment. Although it is possible to obtain friendships and a sense of community at work, such communities tend to be weak as they exist at the discretion of corporate imperatives. Such ties tend to be casual and less supportive than friendships and communities outside of work and although we are spending more time at work, we are not gaining the social capital that is being lost to many people outside of work.

In the current environment, where occupational stability and predictability has decreased, the tendency of workers to focus on their own job is more prevalent, especially in an era of growing competition[122] borne out of performance-based pay and job security. As a result of the efficiency drives of the 1980s and 1990s, a growing number of Americans and British have part-time, temporary or on-call jobs and such jobs tend not to foster a work community in the way that might have been the case in years gone by with the result that the number of Americans satisfied with their jobs fell from 46% to 36% between the mid 1970s and 1992.[122]

The emergence of two career families over the last 25 years has helped to scupper civic disengagement. The commodity of time is less abundant as people have had to be more engaged and invested in their work in order to maintain their standard of living and deflect the growing financial anxieties of the 1970s and 1980s. A greater dependency on increasingly uncertain jobs and a growing need to move around the country in search of work has also contributed to growing isolation between workers and within and between families. What were traditional modes of family life have now been distorted by deregulated labour markets that make it increasingly difficult for many families to even sit down together for meals.[80] The current political culture has created a job market that works to vitiate this shared time and economic pressure, declining real wages and job insecurity have been particularly problematic for those who exist in the lower two-thirds of the income distribution.[122]

Isolation and the Employable Unit

Newt Gingrich and his neoliberal cronies expound family values but there is an irony at the heart of their discourse. In effect, families are not profit making institutions and so their protection means little in the overall scheme of things. Anglo-American capitalism is predicated on isolating people as employable units and this means maximizing any circumstances that enhance this representation and minimizing any circumstances that interfere with it. It is an agenda that is not shared by European capitalism.

Isolation is fundamental, not just from the view of having organized labour and an unrepresentative political process that rewards corporate interests. It is fundamental because it minimizes the elements of the social that interfere with productivity, wealth accumulation and successful consumer demand. Communities and families provide areas for interaction separate to the workplace and such arenas can only impact on the effectiveness of the workplace in this culture of long working weeks.

Furthermore, community and family structures that serve to alleviate the restlessness and dissatisfaction that are the hallmarks of modern consumerism, not to mention offer alternative sources of leisure time, are not effective ways to advance the short-term success of the American business model.

The success in atomizing and isolating the population has been incredible.[79] For example, the town has traditionally represented the centre of communities but their removal at the hands of superstores represents a grave challenge to such communities. Small shops lend a source of social cohesion that is being dismantled around the UK.[102] The number of specialist shops fell by 22% in the UK in the 1990s alone and the number of superstores rose from 457 to 1,102 from the mid 1980s to the mid 1990s (see Chapter 3). The opening of these superstores reduces employment in the area, increases financial strain and diminishes greatly one of the prime meeting centers for social interaction in towns around the country. Practices that lead to superstores being able to drive local business under, such as the use of loss leaders, are allowed in the UK but not in many other countries in the EU.

Frederic Jameson noted that capitalism's alienation of the social is the ultimate threat to human values and communities.[106] The processes and politics of globalization undo social institutions and structures too weak to resist them. As such, individual and community identity are reduced to market logic.[106] Globalization has produced a dissonance that alienates individuals from both global space and from localities with city populations marginalized as the commercialization and privatization of their infrastructure grows apace. Commercial control over increasing amounts of public space, as well as the conversion of the state to a market friendly source of pseudo-governance, has led to poverty, unemployment and altered systems of social support. Moreover, keeping people isolated in a culture that emphasizes individual responsibility for success and failure allows the tacit acceptance of great inconvenience, distress and despair.

This is a system that has grown with Anglo-American capitalism. It is not necessarily the intentional management of a nefarious group of cynics who sit around and plan the best ways to split communities and families (although such individuals are certainly involved). Rather it is a system that has adapted to the demands of the changing laws and political ethos of the countries involved. The process of adaptation is not something that you can always pin down, suffice to say that there has been a generalized, coherent movement in politics, advertizing, business, media and employment that is embracing systems that reinforce and compliment one another. The isolation of people is fundamental to this system since it allows the political elite to create laws and administer advice from the business community that disempowers a greater number of the electorate; it allows the creation of progressively more difficult working conditions, fewer rights, increased social inequality and a growing wealth gap between those who are wealthy and those who are not. It works to provide media representations that explain and excuse such inequality as dispositional traits of citizens and it encourages rampant consumerism in every area of life, including the commodification of childhood and children's education, regardless of the effect this might have.

Privatization, low public investment, growing rates of violent crime, lower civic engagement, deregulation and the disproportional political influence of the business community are the hallmarks of the neoliberal movement. Social isolation and alienation facilitates the representation of people as employment units and so facilitates the neoliberal consensus. When we create computer counseling initiatives, where patients with common mental disorders are treated without any human contact, then we are elevating isolationist tendencies to an artform where disconnection is not only the symptom but the treatment (more on this in Chapter 6).

Globalization and Alienation: Why Is Social Capital Important?

Shareholders and corporate executives are not tied to any given locality and so the consequences of corporate imperatives on local communities are removed. Social cohesion and social capital are a function of shared knowledge, and without constant updating and interaction, they will disintegrate. The removal of public space removes the necessary arena to debate norms and establish values but many of the elites have chosen isolation as their way of life and pay to protect this isolation.[126] However the rest of the population pays the price for their own isolation.

While the effects of low social capital are undoubtedly complex,[127] we know that states in the US that are high in social capital are those where children flourish and are less involved in violent crime. Indeed it is second only to poverty on the effect that it can have on children's lives and living in areas that are characterized by high social capital means that children are less likely to suffer from common mental disorders and behavioural and emotional problems.[122] This is the case even after taking into account all the other usual suspects like poverty, education, inequality and race. Social capital is simply very important to the health of adults and children alike. We know that it is important to children's education because it is higher in areas where parental support for teachers is also higher. If community involvement is high then children will tend to be drawn towards more productive and less alienating forms of leisure activity like television, the effect of which we know can be harmful for many children. Failure to institute a sense of social capital in the local community will undoubtedly mean a failure to expose children to multiple healthy role models, positive norms, informal adult networks and generally limit their opportunity to connect with society as a whole.[122] These children are prey to a variety of social problems like crime, drugs and unemployment. Higher social capital means less murders, it means safer streets, greater peace of mind and greater physical and mental health since such social networks emphasize healthy norms. Indeed in the US, Japan and Scandinavia, the socially disconnected are between two and five times more likely to die from all causes.

Of course this is all very well but if you happen to live in an area of low social capital and high poverty you probably do not have too many options that you can consider with regard to moving to an area of higher social capital. This, however, is not the point. The point is that increasing social capital should be a political aim, an objective for all countries and states because it brings with it a wealth of fundamental improvements in quality of life. The focus on personal control, autonomy and individualism emphasized by our recent concentration on enterprise culture has unrealistically increased our expectations for what we can achieve in isolation. Reasserting social capital as a community objective will help to mend some of the fences bulldozed by recent political and economic machinations.

Summary and Implications

There is little doubt that Anglo-American capitalism is currently the prominent international economic discourse. It is a discourse that is supplanting more social democratic forms of capitalism around the world by way of such institutions as the IMF, the NAFTA, the European Round Table of Industrialists and through other social and political changes over the last 25 years. At the heart of this discourse is a political agenda that seeks to isolate people as units of employment, distinct from the vagaries of community and family life, and so a growing sense of alienation and a reduction in social capital has risen hand in hand with neoliberal ideology in recent years.

This political agenda has had, at its heart, an almost religious reverence for free market fundamentalism, a belief that unregulated markets alone can create and maximize growth for a given economy, a growth that can spread benefits to everyone via trickle down economics and efficient private institutions. The general belief that what is good for a given company is good for the national economy, while being patently untrue,[110] is prevalent in modern commerce and is used to justify political and economic changes that maximize the competitiveness of domestic corporations. At the heart of this agenda is the maximization of shareholder profits and corporate efficiency, regardless of how such an approach dovetails with the democratic, social and environmental imperatives most relevant to the majority of the population. The tenets of neoliberalism are designed to protect wealth and to protect those who have wealth. Such tenets involve the privatization of public sector assets, reduced public investment, reduced employment and tax cuts across the board with the implementation of stealth taxes to move the burden of taxation towards the lower end of the economic spectrum. It involves the movement of power from the political to the private sphere, which means the disempowerment of organized labour and the marginalization of local authorities. It also means an effective 'war on regulation' with the manifestation of weakened government, increased government deregulation initiatives and hence a general corruption of the democratic process. So much so that in Britain there is a British Retail Consortium that boasts of helping to shape government legislation rather than reacting to it.[102]

Such an agenda means automatic cuts to welfare, the stigmatization of welfare recipients and, in the US, the use of welfare sanctions that disproportionately affect states with larger minority populations. It means the growth of a welfare underclass that is no longer necessary as a supply of labour, as would have been the case in previous years. In the UK, such an agenda has led to distortions in the local planning system that allows a disproportionate influence to private developers. Such developers are advantaged to address their own needs and often to the detriment of the local community, a fact particularly prescient in light of the number of property developers on the boards of UK hospital trusts.[91]

We have seen the growing number and influence of superstores in and around towns around the UK. We have seen the growing homogenization of the corporate and political elite such that the public influence on social and economic decisions is growing more and more remote. A renewed focus on individual success at the expense of notions of community or society and the movement of left-wing political parties to the right in search of electoral credibility have reduced the options (or 'choice', the most divine accoutrement of neoliberal acolytes) for democratic political protest.

On an international level, the disproportionate political influence of the business community via the IMF, their clandestine decision-making process and their utter commitment to a 'one size fits all' model of Anglo-American capitalism has had profound consequences for developing countries. The needs of the US business community have led to brash liberalization without the consideration of adequate social and financial institutions and regulatory frameworks. This has led to lower wages, less job protection, cutbacks in health and education spending and increased corruption in 'beneficiary' countries.

This neoliberal political agenda really took off in the US and the UK in the late 1970s and early 1980s and had, in Margaret Thatcher and Ronald Reagan, the ultimate monetarist apostles. But, as one might imagine, such an agenda has not been restricted to the political domain. A number of general social and cultural changes complimented the neoliberal revolution. Some were the result of these political changes and some laid the groundwork for this political revolution to take place. Others simply coevolved. The explosion of school-based marketing and the growing influence of the business community in the curriculum of schools have and will ensure the proliferation of enterprise principles among a new generation. It is certainly not inevitable that a school curriculum influenced by a group of conservative, right-wing, enterprise-oriented businessmen is ideal for the broad ranging education of the future electorate. In the UK, for a £2–3 million donation, the future of our country can be bought by a group of people who do not necessarily have the best interests of the majority of our citizens at heart.

In 1992, the US Committee for Economic Development, an independent, non-profit, non-partisan think tank based in Washington, DC, surmised that 'the government should shift federal policy away from encouraging consumption and towards productive saving and investment'[76] but such a warning has fallen on deaf ears. A decrease in advertizing time constraints and greater exposure to television advertizing has meant that the deleterious effect of this exposure has disproportionately affected the poorer children in society as well as prompting guilt and anguish amongst parents who struggle to provide the products that advertizing tells children are now the basic essentials for their day-to-day existence.

Finally, advantageous reciprocal relationships between politicians, governments and many of the media elite have propagated racially biased, anti-welfare news coverage with the mainstream media defending the social, economic and political agendas of the privileged corporate groups that dominate modern economies and governments.

These recent changes brought about by the neoliberal revolution have emasculated the strength of the family and the community, with social capital disintegrating under the pressure of financial and emotional deprivation. Increases in poverty and deprivation, poor housing conditions, inequality, and decreased health and standard of life are the hallmark social features of this revolution. Reduced occupational protection and security as well as greater dislocation of working communities has led to a rash of poorly paid, temporary or part-time jobs and a growing sense of alienation and social isolation. These social changes have directly contributed to reductions in the quality of life of a growing number of people living in the US and the UK today, with increased illiteracy, decreased health and a greater exposure to crime and aggression contributing to a sense of disillusionment, helplessness and an ebbing sense of hope for the future.

The detrimental social ramifications of the neoliberal revolution have been accompanied by individualist rhetoric that produces representations of poverty as the 'choices' of those who are poor and on welfare, ably supported by a media who disproportionately focus on dispositional, episodic instances of poverty at the expense of societal notions.

So how does the UK Labour government react to the social challenges that the country is currently facing? Who are the personnel used to address the manifest social shortcomings affecting an increasing number of its citizens? George Monbiot[102] highlighted some of the key characters recruited by the current UK government in their quest to win the war against social exclusion. To tackle social exclusion in rural areas, the government decided to use the wisdom of Ewen Cameron, the president of the County Landowner's association and owner of 3,000 acres of Somerset. Stephanie Monk is a vital member of the New Deal task force, a body charged with boosting people's income by moving them off welfare and into work. She is a member of the low pay commission that determines the level of the UK's minimum wage. Stephanie Monk is also the human resources director at Granada Group Plc., a body who appealed against an industrial tribunal's order to reinstate workers who had gone on strike following a decrease in their weekly wage from £140 to £100.[102] We have also had Martin Taylor, the chief executive of Barclays Plc., as chair of the government's tax and benefits task force, a body charged with reducing poverty and welfare dependency. Barclays reduced its workforce by 21,000 from 1987 to 1997. I am sure that with such industrial professionals in place, charged as they are with addressing the structural and political inadequacies that are blighting the lives of so many in the UK, it will only be a matter of time before the problems discussed above evaporate.

However, before jumping to conclude that we are going to hell in a hand cart, these recent political and economic reforms are not unprecedented. The community-destroying global neoliberal economy of recent years is close to that of the late nineteenth century[78,122] and an analysis of economic and political trends shows that a similar deficit in social capital, inequality, degradation, as well as crime was characteristic of the market fundamentalist economy of the late Victorian era. The busy cities of the gilded age were industrial wastelands whose workers were denigrated by stifled competition that led to massive corporations with political power that bode ill for ordinary working people. The difference then was that the US progressives showed manifest civic inventiveness. Small groups mushroomed and became involved in public affairs and sought to bring education to the degraded city inhabitants. Moreover this emphasis on bringing solutions to urban and industrial problems was also a hallmark of the liberal administrations of early twentieth century UK. Today, all major political parties in the UK and the US fight for the political centre ground and there is little organized political or social will to combat the erosion of social democracy. An economy that is progressively exempt from democratic control is not the best prescription for addressing our current economic and social imbalances.[128]

A better example of a country run by economists could not be found than New Zealand between 1984 and 1999.[110] Despite its having experienced the worst economic performance of a rich country in recent years, the performance of such rampant antipodean ultra-neoliberalism failed to influence the political course of its Anglo-American partners, whose brand of capital accumulation continues to displace that of its social democratic European counterpart. The economies of Europe and Asia have come under enormous pressure to dance to the rhythm of the American Business Model.

In 2003, the Bush administration secretly tried to derail the WHO anti-obesity initiative by claiming that there is no link between weight gain and junk food, fast food and soda consumption. They also questioned the link between fruit and vegetable consumption and decreased risk of obesity. The neoliberal world must be a wonderful place to live in, a utopia where everyone benefits from every corporate manifestation of power. We can eat and drink what we like and it will be okay for our health, we can expose our children to forced advertizing for fast food products and they will be healthy and happy. Moreover, they will achieve a fine education; thanks to our altruistic corporate marketers. Hell, why shouldn't we cut corporate tax, these guys are pretty much single-handedly saving America. They are even so kind as to donate funds to America's principle political parties and hence support the greatest democracy in the world. We can sell useless hospitals off and use the land more effectively for houses for our growing population and build more effective hospitals in their place. We can build as many supermarkets and superstores as we can throw a stick at and watch as they single-handedly rejuvenate our communities and increase local trade. Why not cut out the middle man and build properties inside the supermarkets so that we can live there too and then we would barely have to leave these utopian corporate behemoths. The only thing stopping us all from benefiting from these paragons of virtue is the pesky governments and their fastidious regulations. The sooner we can situate governments inside these superstores next to our houses, the better for everyone.

The location of debate has been moved to such an extent that ideas of social justice are often viewed as impossible, simplistic, naïve and harmful. To represent or support such ideas invites marginalization as simplistic liberals with little idea of the machinations of the real world. However such simplistic black and white representations are crude. I own consumer items and love some of them. I have a car, a laptop, a stereo and even watch television. This is not a rant from the dark ages, a Luddite sitting in his house with a transistor radio, determined not to partake in the vagaries of modern living. There are ways to partake in an economy of consumption other than free-market fundamentalism.

The current political, economic and corporate consensus has profound drawbacks that make modern living so much more difficult for so many people than it need be. Thus far I have discussed the social effects of such a political consensus. In the next chapter, I will discuss the profound effect it is having on our mental health.

III: Mental Health

Chapter 5
The Structures of Society and Depression

The previous two chapters have highlighted some of the important political and economic changes that have occurred in the UK and the US in the last 25 years and some of the important effects of those changes. Anglo-American capitalism that focuses on short-term profits at the expense of longer term social and economic gain is currently in the process of supplanting other forms of capitalism, those characterized by capital accumulation that focuses on the benefits of the community as a whole as opposed to a select group of the wealthier members of the community. The Anglo-American model has been ferocious in the speed of its development and the effects in the UK and the US have been profound. This chapter discusses the way that some of the changing social and economic domains relate to the precipitation of mental distress and, specifically, depression.

Depression is now considered to be one of the most serious health issues faced in Europe.[1] In the UK the cost of adult depression is 15.5 billion euros, of which a significant proportion is spent on direct treatment. Moreover, the cost in the US is believed to be around 100 billion euros.[1]

In recent years, there has been a growing understanding of the immense burden that the illness imposes both on individuals and on communities throughout the world, and the disease now represents 4.4% of the total disease burden around the world, in the same range as heart disease.[2] Depressive disorders were estimated to be the leading cause of disability in 1990 and were the fourth leading cause of total global burden of disease. Of even greater importance is the fact that they are predicted to become the second leading cause of global disease burden by 2020.[129] This represents a significant increase and, indeed, a negative prognosis for the world's mental health.

So what is the evidence for the increase in the number of cases of depression? Some will say that an increase in the prevalence of any mental disorder usually results from an improved ability to recognise the given condition or increased public awareness of mental disorders, and hence the likelihood of seeking treatment. While this has undoubtedly been the case in recent years, there is little evidence to suggest that such an increase in the recognition of depression is accountable for the recent rise and the projected rise in the next few years. A review of the evidence strongly suggests that the prevalence (number of people currently depressed) and incidence (number of new cases of depression annually) of major depression as we currently know it are going to increase in the coming years, although it should be noted that such speculation is not conclusive.

A 40-year prospective study with a representative Canadian sample has suggested that the prevalence of depression has increased gradually between 1952 and 1992,[130] and a number of US psychiatrists in the 1970s noted that the rates of depression had greatly increased.[131] A number of authors have supported the contention that there appears to have been an overall increase in the rates of depression and over a number of countries sampled[132–135] with Schor[116] suggesting that the rates of anxiety and depression have soared particularly between the years 1979 and the late 1990s. Indeed, previous research suggests that the notable increase in depression is particularly likely to have taken place following the late 1970s.[136] Furthermore, a number of community surveys in the US, Canada and Sweden have suggested a trend toward an earlier age of onset and an increased rate of people suffering from depression at some point in their lifetime.[131]

Large scale epidemiologic surveys were rarely conducted before the Epidemiologic Catchment Area Programme in 1980 and so much of the information on trends is limited to the past three decades, but a large increase in the number of Americans receiving medication for depression has been found, particularly since the early 1980s and 1990s, although this could be a result of prescribing trends rather than increased prevalence. However, a genuine increase in major depression in recent cohorts has been posited.[14] Furthermore, it has been suggested that depression has increased particularly among younger women over the last 40 years.[130]

With regard to trying to understand the international differences in this increasing prevalence, one encounters a number of problems. Much of the research that has been carried out has tended to provide conflicting results, often as a result of using different methodologies. This could result from different measurement procedures for depression or the social precursors of depression, the use of different instruments, different clinical criteria or different samples, some of which may be more or less representative of the population. Some research has used community samples from the general population while others have focused on general practice participants or participants in psychiatric out-patient settings. Different time periods may have been used with regard to the collection of data and the data may have used different analyses to derive results that are difficult to compare. There is also the problem that there may be different attitudes and perceptions between different countries for taking part in research and this may distort the samples that are being compared.

So although there are a number of studies investigating incidence and prevalence of depression, consistent international differences are difficult to interpret. The studies that have compared different countries with the same research protocol have shown mixed results. Several research projects that have compared depression prevalence have suggested that current rates in the US and UK are higher. Using a measure called the Eurobarometer, the EU research group[137] showed that the UK had a higher prevalence of general mental disorders than Spain, the Netherlands and Portugal. Furthermore, a community sample showed that the UK had a higher

6 month prevalence of major depression than a number of European countries, including Belgium, Germany, the Netherlands and Spain.[138]

Further international research has confirmed that the US has a higher prevalence of depression than a number of other countries.[139,140] However, other projects have provided mixed results regarding the international comparisons with the US and the UK. From the research undertaken thus far, it would be best to conclude that evidence supporting an overall increase in depression over time is unanimous. However, evidence of higher current overall rates of depression in the UK and the US as compared to other countries is inconclusive.[141-143]

There are a number of other possible reasons for this increased prevalence of depression in recent years; what might be referred to as structural factors that create an environment conducive to the development of mental distress and, particularly, depression. As discussed in detail in Chapters 3 and 4, the UK and the US have experienced the largest increases in income inequality of any of the developed market economies over the last 20 years.[144] The enterprise-focused, neoliberal economic and social consensus of recent years has brought about deleterious changes in poverty, social inequality, occupational unpredictability, access to work and working hours. It has also contributed to increased violent and non-violent crime, health problems and decreased social capital. A growing number of us live in a society characterized by unpredictability; where we experience helplessness, hopelessness, decreased social mobility and increased social fragmentation. As discussed in the previous two chapters, there is greater exposure to feelings of desperation and frustration and a reduction in the quality of life of a growing number of the western population, with the international exemplars being the US and the UK.

Only in the 1980s and 1990s has the free market been the dominant social institution.[80] I contend that this radical change in political ethos is a fundamental driving force behind the structural changes that have led to a tangible increase in depression over the last 30 years[116] and the reason why depression is predicted to continue to rise. A cursory glance at much of the social sciences literature could leave the reader with the intuition that the rise in depression prevalence represents a great and complex puzzle of our age, one which needs careful scientific attention to elucidate understanding. I contend that this puzzle has resulted from an excessive focus on the dispositional, personal nature of mental suffering and less so on the enormous political and social changes in recent years.

Depression is not a minor ailment that we just have to put up with. It can be a life-wrecking, hideously painful illness for sufferers and families and one which will soon be the second leading cause of global disease in just over a decade. I believe that much of this considerable suffering is preventable but before discussing how, I need to present my case. Thus far I have discussed the neoliberal political consensus, the increasing influence of Anglo-American capitalism and the egregious social, structural and economic consequences. Now I want to discuss further the link between these consequences and mental ill health, specifically depression.

I expect to see mental health in the UK and the US degenerate quicker than other developed countries around the world that follow models of capitalism less socially destructive than the Anglo-American model. I also expect that, following this initial difference, we will eventually see a reduction in the disparity in depression between many of these other developed countries and the US and the UK as globalization continues apace. Political, social and economic changes are crucial to the physical and mental health of a population, and a sustained movement from an organization characterized by social democracy to one characterized by the rapacious Anglo-American form of capitalism will profoundly influence the propensity for people to develop depression. The situation is worsening but there is no puzzle.

Poverty and Inequality: The Root of All (Mental Health) Evil?

The realities of poverty and inequality can have a number of different meanings for the people who are unfortunate enough to experience them. At the root of such experiences tends to be the unifying concepts of humiliation and a sense of having little or no control over your life. It means feeling trapped in a world where you are bombarded with images of wealth, enterprise and social mobility. It can represent a daily struggle to pay bills, to obtain food and clothes for children. It might mean struggling to find sufficient or permanent work that will allow their families to achieve the minimum quality of life to which they are entitled; a quality of life, the paucity of which constantly drives feelings of guilt and worthlessness. Poverty can mean being exposed to violent crime both inside and outside the family as well as the after-effects of this crime.

It means living in a world that is less and less socially cohesive, where sources of support have gradually dissipated. From the late 1950s until recent times, a pattern of family disintegration, limited social networks and behaviour problems amongst children in schools arose in areas of extreme poverty.[124] Without the finance needed to maintain social and familial relationships, to travel and to entertain, the network of social relations that is so often necessary for support can fall away during difficult times. Indeed half of the families on welfare moved at least once in the previous 2 years, distorting their ability to maintain beneficial family and community ties.[88]

With poverty and inequality comes greater exposure to the most severe life events, events like divorce, unemployment and physical illness. Those in poverty experience substandard and deteriorating housing, peeling paint, decaying properties rife with rodents, crumbling walls and roofs and leaking pipes and usually have little recourse to change these circumstances. Together with inadequate lighting and heating, these aspects of the living environment are precursors of chronic stress and helplessness. It is easy to empathize with the crumbling self-esteem of people who have to exist in a daily atmosphere of decay and filth while constantly exposed to the lifestyles of the wealthy. When we add feelings of limited political power, poorer standards of education and perceptions of inadequate access to police protection, we realize that the increase in poverty and inequality in the US and the UK in recent years has increased the number of families constantly searching for a better life but with ever diminishing opportunities to do so.

Poverty means worrying not only about yourself but about your children who are more likely to be assaulted, murdered, arrested, victimized, unemployed and dropout of school than children from families not in poverty. The experience of taking welfare itself is manifestly stigmatizing, especially so in the US where feelings of humiliation and degradation are prompted by the status of welfare-user in a culture that overwhelmingly blames poverty on the poor. Low expectations of success, deficits in social skills and unstable family environments combine to contribute to the often lasting nature of poverty from which so many people simply do not believe that they can escape.

Some readers may not recognize the lifestyle descriptions above or believe that they have been cribbed from a melodramatic Victorian novel charting the lifestyle of the poor creatures who were desperately trying to avoid the pull of the workhouse. However, these experiences are very real for a growing number of people in the US and the UK. The bottom line is that living in poverty exposes people to many sources of chronic, long-term stress and removes many of the very sources of support that they need to challenge and overcome these stresses. Perhaps not surprisingly, an analysis of the literature on stress and mental health provides strong evidence that the experience of poverty and of being poor contributes significantly to reductions in mental health and particularly to increased depression. The aggregate impact of poverty on the population is likely to be considerable.[145]

The news that poverty or social exclusion is related to mental health problems is not necessarily new with regards to policy directives.[146] Documents published by the UK Department of Health in 1997 acknowledged such a relationship. The problem is that the strategy and policy documents published since then have tended to focus on mental health as the driving force behind social exclusion rather than the other way around. There is little doubt that the relationship between poverty and depression is complex and that causation could indeed be bidirectional. However, little reliable evidence exists that shows reverse causation, that is, depression as the driving force behind social exclusion and poverty.[144,146,147]. What is often referred to as the 'downward drift' hypothesis, in which people with mental illness will move down the social class gradient, is simply not borne out by the data.

However, some authors[144] have suggested that inequality could have dire consequences for the mental health of the population and a number of different studies, with different kinds of measurements and samples, have shown this to be the case. The British Office of Population Censuses and Surveys found higher rates of depression and anxiety among men and women with lower educational qualifications and in lower occupational groups.[148] Furthermore, people living in long-term economic hardship and financial strain have been shown to be more likely to be suffering from clinical depression than those not exposed to such long term hardship.[146,149] Indeed, the median rate of psychological disturbance in US community studies tends to be 36% in the lowest social class, whereas in the highest social class this figure drops to 9% and the authors noted that social factors were often chronic and persistent.[150]

There is a considerable and growing literature that shows that poverty and economic deprivation is associated with an increased prevalence of mental disorders, including not only depression and anxiety but also substance abuse[71,122,123,131,151–153], with depressed groups suffering from greater economic deprivation than healthy controls.[71] Common mental disorders like depression and anxiety have been shown to be associated with low material standard of living within all occupational strata, and Weich and Lewis[65] showed that a poor material standard of living accounted for nearly 25% of prevalent cases of common mental disorder.

Between 1971 and 1998 a review of the literature that looked at 51 separate studies across different countries and using different methodologies concluded that differences in rates of depression as a result of socioeconomic status were a robust international phenomenon. Rates of depression were significantly greater in the highest socioeconomic groups than in the lowest socioeconomic groups in the UK, the US, France, Germany, New Zealand, Germany and Sweden. Furthermore, the research showed that those studies undertaken in North America had a steeper gradient than the others. That is, the difference in rates of depression was most pronounced between the socioeconomic groups in North America.[154] The research in the West that has shown that rates of depression are significantly higher in low socioeconomic status areas than high socioeconomic status areas has also been replicated in a small number of studies in developing countries.[124]

It has been shown that poverty not only predicts current risk of depression but that it predicts depression in the future. Data from the New Haven Epidemiologic Catchment Area study showed that poverty at first contact predicted a doubling of the risk of a major depressive episode.[145] Financial strain appears to be the critical mediator behind the greater depression associated with unemployment[155] and the experience of being in debt to one or more companies in the last year makes someone significantly more likely to experience poor mental health. It has been suggested that the profound fear of eviction and impending homelessness associated with falling into mortgage arrears has led to nearly 80% of such people suffering from mental disorder.[146]

Admission rates to psychiatric wards have also been shown to be associated with poverty. Platt and colleagues[123] noted that, compared to more affluent electoral wards, admission rates to psychiatric units were six times higher in the two most deprived electoral wards. Using a number of different measures, it has also been shown that deprivation is related to neurotic disorder, of which depression and anxiety are important components. People with no access to a car, used as a proxy for relative deprivation, were considerably more likely to be at increased risk of neurotic disorder than those with access to two or more cars. Furthermore, people who rented their homes were also at increased risk although it should be noted that the authors found no independent association between relative deprivation and educational attainment.[144,152] Work has also shown that, not only is the experience of being poor important to mental health and depression, but feeling poor is also associated with a higher risk of common mental disorders like anxiety and depression.[146] Those who felt poor all of the time reported feeling isolated and more than half reported feeling depressed. Even among those who were poor, the subjective experience of feeling poor was a risk factor for greater common mental disorders, although it should be stressed that the objective measure of actually being poor was still more associated with common mental disorders.

The growth in single parents over recent years has had a significant effect on mental health and depression. This is particularly important when we bear in mind that the number of single parent families grew from 8% in 1971 to 21% in 1992.[145] Single parents are more likely to suffer from depression than any other demographic, some of which is directly attributable to the poverty and social exclusion often related to the experience of being a single parent. That said, the actual burden of parenting is greater in single parent households than in two parent households and mental ill-health has been shown to be related to single parenthood even after taking poverty into account.[146]

Research carried out on a cross section of residents of New York City showed that neighbourhood social disorganization was associated with depressive symptoms and that living in a socio-economically deprived area is associated with the presence of depression.[156] Indeed, poor housing, particularly housing characterized by high rise dwelling and damp and mould, has been shown to be associated with mental health and psychiatric consultation.[123] It has also been shown that those in social housing are more likely to suffer poor mental health than owner occupiers and that this impact of poor housing would appear to be greater for women than for men.[146]

To further implicate the importance of the neighbourhood in the rates of depression, work which has monitored the changes in depression in a group who change neighbourhoods has shown interesting results. A recent housing voucher experiment in the US showed that the rates of depression decreased in women and children who moved from high poverty urban neighbourhoods to low poverty suburban neighbourhoods.[157]

This influence of different indices of economic deprivation has been shown to extend to specific aspects of the experience of suffering from depression. For instance, a number of authors have shown that financial hardship and lower socioeconomic status have been shown to be associated with longer, more chronic episodes of depression and thus longevity of suffering.[145,158] Once depressed, people of lower socioeconomic status were shown to be over two times as likely to stay depressed than those from a higher socioeconomic status.[154] It has been suggested that socioeconomic status and financial strain, as well as being associated with onset of a depressive episode,[65] actually delay recovery from mental illness.[65,152] We know that low income patients, with less knowledge of treatments for depression and those with lower education, are less likely to prefer active treatment[159] and this could be one of the factors driving this greater chronicity in the poor.

How Important is Childhood Poverty?

Much of the research that has been carried out thus far has tended to focus on the relationship between adult poverty, deprivation and depression, but research suggests that the associations found above also hold for children. It appears that children from poorer families have poorer academic achievement, nutritional status and social development than more advantaged children.[160] They tend to have more mental health problems generally, and higher rates of depression specifically, than non-poor children, and those children with an early history of persistent poverty had higher levels of depression over the 5 years that they were examined, regardless of their subsequent experience of poverty.[161] Simply put, it appears that early economic disadvantage has long term effects on mental health. This long term effect of consistent poverty during the first five years of a child's life also influences the child's depression during adolescence and this effect is independent of the mental health status of the child's mother.[162]

Although the vast majority of research findings suggest a causal association between poverty, deprivation and depression, not all of the research in the field supports such an assertion and some inconsistencies have been found between the different measures of income inequality used by different researchers.[149,163] Some work has found that socioeconomic status is more powerfully related to anxiety disorders than depression[164] and recent research has failed to confirm evidence to support the contention that socioeconomic adversity is associated with the maintenance of depression.[165] However, such evidence is very much in a minority and could have arisen from methodological differences regarding the units of geography used to define poorer areas. It could also be due to a growing experience of financial strain, and hence depression, among a broad socioeconomic spectrum of neighbourhoods. Overall though, the evidence overwhelmingly corroborates a strong relationship between poverty, social deprivation and mental health status, particularly depression, and this relationship is unlikely to result from reverse causality. Poverty and financial strain increase the likelihood of a person suffering from depression.

Life Events: Generations of Depression

While so far we have focused on poverty and financial strain, there has also been a growing number of studies that have confirmed the importance of other stressful and difficult life events, many of which are related to issues of material deprivation. Such life experiences as bereavement, moving house, social alienation, employment difficulties, the breakdown of a relationship and suffering a long-term or debilitating illness have been considered to be causes of depression.[122,162,166] Indeed, the strongest relationship between life events and the onset of depression has been shown to be between threatening and undesirable events and depression onset.[122,123] Longer duration of depression appears to be associated with marital difficulties or widowhood, with a shorter duration of illness associated with lifetime trauma.[145,167]

The turmoil produced by a severe life event can represent a loss of routine as much as the actual crisis. Work on a group of women from London showed that events with a long term rather than a short term threat have a causal role in depression and that nearly half of the women with depression experienced a severe event of causal importance. This event was usually related to loss and it was shown that multiple unrelated severe events increased the risk of depression. Long term difficulties have also been shown to be of some importance since they are three times as common in depressed women than in non-depressed women. Moreover, working class women with children at home are four times as likely to develop depression and this greater probability was considered to result from their greater chance of experiencing provoking factors.[10]

The Stress of Child Adversity and Depression

The relationship between stressful and difficult life events in childhood and depression appears to be particularly important. A factor that significantly predicts depression that lasts more than 12 months is childhood adversity, with factors such as parental indifference, lack of parental warmth, inconsistent parental rearing attitudes, parental relationship difficulties, family violence and interpersonal problems being of particular importance.[20,30,162] Child abuse and depression are closely linked with research suggesting that a considerable number of adults suffering from depression have experienced emotional deprivation in infanthood, had parents who had experienced emotional deprivation, had been physically or emotionally abused or had been the victims of sexual abuse or incest.[17] Moreover, this history of serious childhood physical abuse has been shown to differ between depressed and non-depressed controls.[71] The feeling of helplessness and unpredictability associated with such abuse is particularly important with regard to the development of a predisposition to depression.

So how do these developmental factors actually influence adult mental health? It has been assumed that the psychosocial developmental factors discussed above create a vulnerability that predisposes these people by possibly lowering the threshold to a wide range of triggering factors such as life stresses and strains or physical illness. It could be that they specifically lower the threshold to triggers especially salient to the experience of the person and that may have particular importance with regard to the experiences they suffered as children.[16] Such theories tie in with the idea of learned helplessness discussed in Chapter 1. The 'lock and key' theory of depression suggests that the triggering events in adulthood may not necessarily relate logically to childhood difficulties. For instance, a debilitating physical illness in adulthood may mean that the sufferer experiences a lack of control and predictability over the events in their life, or a sense of hopelessness, feelings that they may also have experienced in response to sexual or physical abuse as a child. Moreover, the experience of such feelings may be particularly likely to lead to depression in this particular person. Of course, it is perfectly reasonable to suggest that such theories rely on retrospective interpretation of childhood events that may be distorted, and hence fundamentally inaccurate, but whether this is true or not does not denigrate the robust association between childhood abuse and depression.

There has also been work that suggests a physiological rationale for the relationship between childhood abuse and other childhood difficulties, and an adult predisposition to develop depression. Early life difficulties have been associated with robust abnormalities in the Hypothalamic Pituitary Axis (HPA), an important system in the body involved in the regulation of stress via parts of the brain called the hippocampus and prefrontal cortex.[20] It has been suggested that adrenocortical responses (that is, those involved in the regulation of stress hormones) may develop differently depending on the exposure to stressful childhood events (and indeed, ongoing stress in adulthood). Chronic over-stimulation of the HPA stress response system is likely to be toxic to hippocampal neurons and there certainly appears to be evidence that lower volumes of hippocampal neurons exist in depressed patients as compared to controls.[19] Studies have confirmed that this happens early in the course of depression or may precede the onset of the illness. We know that decreased hippocampal volume is found in people with major depression[20] and that high levels of the stress hormone cortisol are related to more severe depressions.[168] The effects of such early damage to the brain may not appear until several years after the damage has occurred and so the deleterious effects of chronic childhood distress and abuse may not be obvious until adulthood where they take the form of a predisposition toward depression. Indeed, the association between depression and decreased hippocampal volume exists even after recovery and so may be related to the probability of relapse and recurrence.

So what does this actually mean? Well the difficulties experienced by these children, and the associated physiological changes that may in some way predispose them to the development of depression, could lead to an increased likelihood of the illness being transmitted through generations within specific economic groups in society. For instance, it has been shown that poor women, and especially those with young children, are more likely to experience psychological problems than wealthier women. It has been suggested that maternal depression is associated with language and cognitive problems, insecure parental attachment, difficulties in social interaction and behavioural problems.[160] Some authors have suggested that mothers who are depressed are less responsive to their children, more helpless, critical, hostile, less warm and nurturing and less autonomous.[17,162] They are considered to be generally less competent and it is possible that the social and economic stressors of poverty affect children and adolescents indirectly through disruptions in their relationship with a struggling parent. As well as being at a higher risk of developing depression,[125,162] these children of depressed parents are considered to be at a higher risk of developing conduct problems, failure at school[161] and anxiety. Indeed, in some parents with depression this propensity for childhood depression was very strong. Sixty-four percent of depressed children had a depressed mother whereas 15% of non-depressed children were found to have depressed mothers.[17] Of course, it should be noted that we cannot rule out the reverse relationship, that anxious and depressed children are capable of inducing mental health problems in parents and so there could be an element of bidirectional influence involved.

The literature on the relationship between parental depression and childhood depression and other difficulties is robust and an understanding of the psychological and social factors is undoubtedly key but one cannot rule out the genetic transfer of propensities for illness, especially when keeping in mind the research outlined in Chapter 1 that provided evidence for a gene/environment interaction. The fact that depression is a generational issue means that there is a greater transfer of emotional difficulties in certain groups in society. The experience of living with a depressed parent is more common for poor children, and disenfranchised, distressed parents exposed to psychological and social stressors are more likely to be depressed and to negatively affect the mental health of their children. Through the direct physical and emotional consequences of deprivation, and the indirect consequences of severe difficulties in the parent–child relationship, risk factors can accumulate over time as many children struggle with the hardships of poverty.[169] As such, depression has a considerably greater likelihood of being promulgated through generations of families in society that are more likely to be exposed to the stresses and strains that are known to be risk factors for depression. Indeed, this generational transfer may be one of the reasons behind the continued increase in the prevalence of the disease. As more people are exposed to the precipitating factors that predict depression, a greater number of people are affected because not only the adults, but their children, are at greater risk of developing depression in the future. When we factor into this scenario the fact that experiencing depression is itself a risk factor for future episodes of depression, then we have a recipe for a continued increase in prevalence in the years to come.

Urban Living, Isolation and Depression

It would be well short of a revelation to point out that urbanization can, and has, led to separation among the occupational, familial and institutional aspects of our everyday life in the West. Indeed, social commentators back in the early part of the twentieth century were lamenting the poor social integration, alienation and social withdrawal that were such strong features of urban living.[124] Fast-forward to 2005 and Trevor Phillips, the Chairman of the UK Commission for Racial Equality, warned that the July 7th London transport bombings exposed a nightmare of racial segregation, with some city districts becoming fully fledged ghettos.[170]

One of the main features of capitalism is an increase in urbanization. However, it is not necessarily urbanization per se that is proving harmful to the people who live in our big cities. I am not going to preach that a return to a simple life in the fields is a solution for the mental health problems that we face in the coming years.

Rather, it is the type of urbanization that is contributing to an increase in behavioural disturbance, a breakdown of the family unit and increased depression and anxiety among the urban population.[128] This kind of urbanization is closely related to poverty and has led increasingly to a profound increase in social isolation, urban crowding, poor working conditions, underemployment, chronic hunger, limited education and gender discrimination. It has also facilitated housing problems, child-rearing difficulties, reduced personal security, higher levels of violence and an over-crowded physical environment. An increase in single-parent households and for many, the profound and chronic stress associated with modern urban living has played a part in the increased incidence of depression. For instance, with increasing levels of urbanization, the incidence of depression rose between 12 and 20%, as compared to a group least exposed to urban living.[12] A review of studies on mental disorders in urban populations showed that 80% of research reported a higher frequency of mental disorder in urban than in rural populations[124] and some authors have specifically implicated low income and structural housing problems as the prominent factors that were associated with the prevalence of depression and anxiety.[163] Kessler and colleagues[14] showed that people living in rural areas have a 40% lower probability of experiencing multiple mental disorders than those living in urban areas. Escalating rates of depression and anxiety have been shown to be a principle feature of these differences and work in Taiwan has shown that the rapid industrial changes, urbanization and related social changes between the 1940s and 1980s were associated with increasing levels of depression.[124]

However, the differences found thus far have not only been shown between urban and rural populations. Further research that has looked at differences between urban and suburban areas has suggested that urban living may be more likely to predispose its citizens to major depression, although it has been noted that the findings on the issue are not uniform.[134,171]

The built environment of the area that people live in has been shown to be important with regard to mental health. People living in poorer neighbourhoods (as measured by built environment) were between 29 and 58% more likely to report depression in the previous 6 months and 36–64% more likely to report depression over their lifetime than the neighbourhoods characterized by a better built environment.[156] The prevalence of depression was associated with independently rated features of the built environment, regardless of the socio-economic status and internal characteristics of the homes of the respondents. This suggests that it is not only income-related factors but other elements of poverty that are closely related to the prevalence of depression in a given area and social environmental difficulties like graffiti, vandalism, traffic and pollution and crime could play a prominent role.[163] This is of particular interest since, with regards to crime, the 50 years up to 1987 saw violent crime in England and Wales rise at an unprecedented rate[83] and serious crimes known to the police in England leapt from 1.6 million in 1970 to 2.8 million barely 10 years later.[80]

Belying former UK Home Secretary Douglas Hurd's statement that 'prison is an expensive way of making bad people worse', this change in the number of crimes has led to incarceration rates of more than one in a thousand in the UK and approaching one in a hundred in the US,[80] and such figures directly contribute to the anxieties and difficulties associated with single parenthood. Black people are now approximately seven times more likely than whites to be imprisoned and so, together with their greater likelihood of living in poverty, are suffering disproportionately from the adverse mental health consequences associated with incarceration and crime both on the victims and on the families of the perpetrators. As touched upon earlier, the greater insecurity and anxiety of people in urban environments now acts as a profound source of chronic distress and has further contributed to civic isolationism, as 28% of the US population now live in privately guarded buildings or housing developments.

Alienation, Social Support and Depression

This growing sense of social isolation is particularly important since depression and other mental disorders cannot be dissociated from the environmental contexts that frame our everyday lives. The post-war expansion in housing led to young families being placed in isolated blocks of flats with the associated disruption to community and family networks. As discussed in the previous chapter, social capital, the sense of community and cohesion within a given neighbourhood, is gaining importance in social policy and public health.[172] The social capital of an area is important in a number of ways that were outlined in the previous chapter and the positive effects of community integration should not be underestimated. Indeed, the more integrated we are with our communities, the less likely we are to experience a whole range of serious illnesses.

Social networks provide tangible health assistance as well as reinforcing healthy modes of behaviour. However, it is not only physical health problems that benefit from high social capital. Social capital has a particular bearing on mental health and men in low social capital areas are nearly twice likely to show psychiatric morbidity than those in the highest social capital area.[172] It has been shown to be significantly associated with depression in particular.[122] Higher rates of depression have been found in people who report feelings of isolation over the previous 12 months as a result of the difficulties related to the cost and availability of transport, paid work, issues related to childcare and being unable to socialize with friends and family.[146] The size of a person's social network is important, with larger social networks being associated with better mental health.[173] The size of a person's primary group (the social support network) is significantly smaller in psychiatric outpatients than community controls.[135] Over the years some of the leading theorists on suicide, like Emile Durkheim and Roy Baumeister, have reiterated the importance of poor social integration as a precipitating factor in both negative mood and suicide.[23,55]

This progressive and continued spatial segregation and a growing sense of alienation from members of extended families and communities creates a sense of distress in many but, as importantly, it removes a key resource that protects against the onset and exacerbation of depression. Social support is profoundly important with regard to coping with everyday challenges and strong interpersonal ties protect people from becoming distressed. Social interaction is not the same as social support and strong, supportive relationships are often needed to reduce feelings of helplessness and low self regard, to reduce the impact of what can often seem like crushing life events. The feeling of not being isolated, of experiencing a rich support network, can be of great help for many people as they move through difficult times.[174]

Social networks are particularly important with regard to protecting against depression.[175,176] Women with a close and confiding relationship with their partner are at a lower risk of depression than others without this relationship facility[146] and in men, a source of confiding emotional support has also been shown to have a positive effect on mental health.[177] The importance of the social sphere was highlighted in a 12 month follow-up study that showed that people with some, moderate or severe social disability were at greater risk for the development of depression.[178] Social support is so crucial that elevated symptoms of depression appear as the most frequent and consistent outcome of poor social support.[175] Indeed, a lack of social support predicts not only the onset of depression, but a longer episode of depression, and the quality of social support that a person experiences and the importance of caring from friends and family was felt by many to be 'the difference between getting through the illness and not'.[3,167,179]

Work with depressed participants has shown that being married independently predicted recovery from depression[158,180] and relationship quality is of great relevance since dissatisfied spouses are nearly three times more likely than satisfied spouses to develop an episode of major depression, regardless of demographic status or lifetime history of depression.[177,181] The importance of relationship status was highlighted by work that showed that being separated or divorced has been shown to predict a greater likelihood of developing depression.[178]

Single mothers who report low social support are most at risk from the onset of depression. This is particularly relevant since they are at the greatest risk of experiencing the kind of severe life events that are likely to precipitate depression in the first instance.[146] Indeed, the combination of low social support together with a low standard of living substantially increases the likelihood of psychological distress[16,146,177] and support from family members, and other social networks has been shown to be associated with reduced risk of depression in low income women specifically.[89]

There have also been suggestions that cultures that are more characterized by the interdependent collective are less likely to express individually oriented statements of dysphoria.[182] However, whether such networks are responsible for lower symptoms or whether they are responsible for a lower likelihood of expressing these symptoms has been debated.

As with poverty, the issue of cause and effect is important since it would be feasible to expect that depression itself would act to diminish social ties and social support as well as the alternative, but results indicate that social support is far more likely to be the driving force behind depression and marital dissolution is far more likely to be a cause than a consequence of depression.[55]

So far I have discussed the relationship between depression, poverty and the reductions in social capital associated with progressive urbanization, but of course poverty and the development and maintenance of social networks are related. A lack of income can seriously impinge upon the possibilities for social network development and integration[183] and such a lack of social integration that results from being unable to finance sociality will lead to greater isolation and feelings of alienation. If you cannot afford to visit malls, shops, own phonecards or mobile phones and cannot afford the clothing with which to subjectively make yourself respectable, then such community and family ties can easily drift. Feeling like a second class citizen because you are unable to exist at the same consumer level as members of your close network can lead to a distancing of people from those around them and such considerations are more common than many people realize. Social capital and social support both influence mental health status, and considerable evidence suggests that having less social support with which to cope with the increased stresses and strains that urban living creates is fundamental to mental health and depression. Reduced housing quality and greater social isolation are profound problems that increase the risk for developing depression and decrease the likelihood of recovering from depression and these factors are endemic in urban environments.

Occupation

So far I have discussed the importance of poverty and social support/social capital with regard to depression and have hopefully shown just how important these factors are when it comes to developing and recovering from an episode of the illness. One further area closely related to poverty and standard of material living and which, like poverty, inequality and social capital, is radically changing as a result of the current political and economic consensus, is that of employment and the different factors related to employment. As touched upon in the last chapter, one of the key features of globalization has been the way that employers have been able to adopt a more flexible approach to their workforce. While this has considerable benefits for a number of multinational and national corporations seeking to increase economic efficiency, the result for the majority of employees has been less security of employment, reduced benefits and rights for workers and a growth in the number of casual, temporary and part-time staff. It has also meant a reduction in the power of organized labour and a general increase in employee apprehension and lack of control over the future.

Between 1969 and 1987 the fraction of the labour force who were working part-time but desired full-time work increased more than seven times.[85] The loss of jobs in the 1980s' manufacturing sector in the US and the UK put a premium on schemes such as adjustment programmes and training programmes, which have been shown to significantly lower rates of unemployment and income loss and mean that workers suffer fewer of the social difficulties associated with long-term unemployment. However, in the US, companies that take active participation in readjustment programmes and provide adequate advance notice of job termination tend to be the exception rather than the rule.[90] Despite the obvious benefits of such programmes and of advance notice, a succession of US administrations have, in their desire to highlight their corporate credentials, tried wherever possible to reduce the burden on companies when it comes to terminating the employment of their workers.

The number of people who have been excluded from access to work in the west has been growing in recent years regardless of strong economic performances and growth in these countries.[80] The recent strong economic growth in the US has, under current labour market conditions, resulted in a great growth in low paid female work in the service, food and retail sectors but has simply failed to create jobs that are moving people out of poverty.[125] The jobs created are characterized by a culture that is bereft of hope, upward mobility or adequate benefits.

While the nature of employment has changed in recent years, the actual time spent at work has steadily increased over the same period. Men were working nearly 100 hours more per year in 1987 than in 1969 and the need to hold down two jobs in order to pay off debts and meet household expenses has become a common occurrence.[85] Most working mothers are effectively holding down two jobs if we factor in the burden of cleaning, child care, laundry and housework. A survey in Boston showed that most employed mothers average over 80 hours of work if employment, childcare and housework are amalgamated[85]. Maintaining the balance between work and family has become more and more difficult and has become a source of chronic stress as leisure time, and the time spent with children and with partners/spouses, declines in order to provide a livable income. Relationship satisfaction and parental guidance for children falls by the wayside as financial imperatives take precedence. For many, the strain associated with the changes in the employment environment, and the social and financial results of such changes, can be immense.

It is known that employers are significantly affected by mental illness and depression in particular. Depression has been linked to diminished productivity, increased absence through sickness, disability and lower morale,[152,184] with research suggesting that the costs of depression amounted to many billions of dollars. When we consider this, and that depression and anxiety account for more than one third of days lost from work,[65] it is clear that it is not sufferers and their families alone who exist at the sharp end of the illness. So bearing this in mind, one might think it paradoxical that employment practices and cultures would play a role in the precipitation and reduced recovery from depression. However, the literature suggests that this is certainly the case and that recent changes to employment culture in the west will exacerbate an already growing problem.

The Association Between Employment and Depression

In 1999, the UK Poverty and Social Exclusion Survey confirmed previous findings that one of the key factors affecting mental health is the level and status of employment.[146] Basically, the role that people have can fundamentally affect their mental health and research suggests that the characteristics of people's work contribute toward well-being and depression more than social mobility.[177] Having a variety of tasks in a job, having a greater degree of control over work and having greater opportunity to use occupational skills were associated with low scores in depression and anxiety. This finding has been confirmed by other authors[123] who have noted a complexity in the issue of job variety. Having multiple roles within a job is protective of mental health problems when the employment is reasonably rewarded but less so when it is not. Moreover, the feeling of being undermined at work has also been shown to be important to the psychological health of a great many workers.[3] The Whitehall study in the UK was constructed to investigate the causes of social gradients in mental health and, as regards employment, confirmed that work demands, control and support at work are protective of future psychiatric morbidity,[173] regardless of previous psychiatric disorder. Another key factor that has been found in relation to mental health and employment is the double burden of paid and unpaid work, as is experienced by many women.[146]

The experience of unemployment, especially long-term unemployment, is undoubtedly a risk factor for depression and other mental health problems and this has been confirmed in a number of studies.[122,123,146,155,177,185] Those defined as unemployed are most likely to suffer high levels of all psychiatric disorders[146] and both men and women are at greater risk of developing depression when they have experienced unemployment for more than 12 months in the last 10 years. Greater casual and temporary work means more unemployment in between these shorter periods of employment and this can lead to a number of difficulties.

Again the issue of reverse causality arises in any research that analyses associations between variables but, as with previous sources of mental health distress, research suggests that unemployment is more likely to predate the onset of depression than the other way around.[123,186–188]

As mentioned in the previous chapter, the continued emphasis on the work ethic has led to employment status gaining a profound sense of importance in and of itself, regardless of the alleviation of financial strain that it provides. However, the alleviation of financial strain is of critical importance since some believe that financial strain is the crucial mediator between unemployment and depression.[155] Paid work can help people to avoid unstructured time and help to raise self-esteem whilst obviously avoiding the stigma attached to unemployment and welfare. The loss of paid work also leads to the loss of valued personal relationships, of personal identity or at least a personal identity that the sufferer is comfortable with. Employment status can also affect mental health via destructive relationship patterns and mental health problems in spouses.[145,175] The financial strain that affects those with employment difficulties has also been shown to increase the symptoms of depression in partners and this can impinge on their ability to provide a given level of support to their partner.

The meaningful goals, ambitions and plans for the future can dissipate along with the ability to act as provider for the family and a sense of personal control can become a thing of the past. Long-term, uncontrollable unemployment is positively predictive of depression for a number of reasons but the removal of hope is one of the most important. The hope that one can be reintegrated into society via paid employment can easily diminish as the duration of unemployment increases, and such a sense of hopelessness and helplessness can create a chronic strain and remove the motivation needed to actually escape these aversive circumstances. Subsequent depression robs the sufferer of the ability and emotional strength to find new employment and can lead to what feels like a 'downward spiral'.

Recent changes in employment culture are likely to have exposed a generation and their families to a higher likelihood of becoming depressed. This is especially damaging because nothing precipitates depression like previous depression. Those who have suffered depression are more likely to suffer from recurrent future depression when faced with further challenges and so a cultural downward spiral exists with the result of ever increasing levels of depression. Indeed, this is what we are witnessing. With regard to reducing social exclusion and addressing the physical and mental health of the populous, one of the current tactics of the UK government is to enrol as many people as possible into the labour market.[146] While this may seem initially promising, it should be borne in mind that such an imperative provides a justification for returning many to lower paid jobs with greater uncertainty, less control at work and reduced employee benefits.

The Gender 'Puzzle'

There are sex differences in depression that have been highlighted by countless studies across different clinical groups, cultures and countries. If you are a woman, you are two times as likely to be depressed as compared to men, a rate that is increasing.[184] To try to understand this difference is far from straightforward as we have to fully appreciate the extent of the biological, economic, occupational and cultural norms that differ between the sexes. We have to better understand our representations of men and women and the different pressures to which they are exposed. This is an enormously complex area because sex roles and responsibilities vary hugely between different generations and cultures. However, in recent years a growing literature has suggested that the social pressures that many women face play a significant role in the differences in depression between men and women. Indeed, the general absence of sex differences in genetic research showing the interaction of the 5HT transporter alleles and environmental stressors has led some authors to speculate that the increased prevalence of mood disorders in women may be related to factors other than genetic influence.

The higher rate of depression in women may well reflect the fact that they are generally subject to more stressful life events, chronic difficulties, discrimination and victimization.[133] Western women have experienced a long history of culturally enforced limitations regarding their capacity to express themselves in society through occupational, educational, political and economic means. While recent history suggests greater freedom and opportunities for women, opportunities in the west are significantly skewed in favour of men. From a female perspective, men still control 99% of the world's resources and this disparity has resulted in women operating as second class citizens in a number of cultural domains. For instance, with regard to jobs, there still exists outright discrimination in hiring, prospects for internal promotion and wages paid to women. Lower wages are generally paid to the female workforce, often for carrying out the same work as male colleagues and this disparity in wages is often considerable. For instance in the US women still make 72 cents for every dollar made by men.[88] This finding has been echoed in the UK.[75]

By 1990 two-thirds of married women in the United States were participants in the paid labour market.[85] Working mothers effectively hold down two jobs when one adds laundry, cleaning, housework and the many tasks involved in childcare to their paid employment.[85] Women meet the requirements of a cheap workforce and weak laws protecting workers has allowed this practice to continue.[152]

Single parenting is also an important issue. The divorce law reform act of 1969 made it easier for couples to divorce and during the 1980s there were 160,000 UK divorce decrees every year. This meant a heavy increase in largely female single parents. When we consider single working mothers who suffer from this pay disparity, while also organizing childcare, one can imagine the cumulative stresses that many modern single working women encounter and these have been shown to impact on their mental health.[146] High levels of depressive symptoms are common among those with low incomes generally, but this is especially the case with mothers with young children. Indeed, 40% of African-American mothers in the US have reported symptoms that suggest a diagnosis of depression.[89] Rates of major depression in low-income mothers are about twice as high as the general population of women, suggesting that this combination of being female and of low income creates a particularly high risk population.[71,89,123] The onset of depression has been linked with the experience of entrapping or humiliating life events and these are more common in women who experience financial strain. Indeed, single mothers are considered to be twice as likely to experience entrapment or humiliation as mothers with partners and the delinquent behaviour of children features prominently.[145]

As mentioned earlier, experiencing poverty can remove the facility to fulfill important and desired social roles as well as expose people to the disabling stigma that many welfare recipients feel. Since many of these women take the majority of the responsibility for childcare duties, they may also be more affected by feelings of guilt and inadequacy at being a 'bad parent' and a poor provider since they are exposed to the perceived financial deficiencies that their children experience. This is particularly important when their children are increasingly exposed to the consumer possibilities presented by television advertising. They may also feel disproportionate guilt associated with not being able to spend a given amount of time with their children as they struggle to balance employment, household chores and childcare. There are strong cultural precedents for women with regards to the time they should spend with their children and transgressing upon these precedents can lead to distress in many women. In conjunction, it has been suggested that poorer women with children have fewer opportunities for contact with friends and family due to their isolated locations on peripheral estates.[123]

Institutionalized Depression for the Modern Woman

The structure of institutions within society is important. Gender-based structural oppression can include social controls over women's sexuality, social pressure to organize their bodies in increasingly unrealistic shapes, rights within a marriage, reproductive rights and violence against women. We know that economic autonomy, employment, earnings and reproductive rights are significantly related to women's depression[157] and we also know that for those who are married, a lower status within marriage is considered to increase their vulnerability to mental health problems.[175]

Although not a hard and fast rule for everyone, there is a cultural sanction for men to channel their distress outward through violence or alcohol use. Women have traditionally been compelled to internalize their responses to distress and their greater depression and anxiety may be a response, not only to the greater stresses and difficulties that they experience, but from the facility that they have to respond to that distress. That is not to apportion responsibility for the distress to the women as a result of their coping styles. This is less likely to be a result of genetic or 'natural' biological factors than responses to the social dominance hierarchies to which they are exposed. Women inhabit lesser positions of power and by that I mean power as a characteristic of relationships between people and between people and institutions. Those who exist in lower positions of power have little opportunity to react to, or ameliorate, the circumstances to which they are exposed, often from those in positions of dominance.

In the context of a relationship or a marriage, this can result from a woman who is economically dependent on a dominant partner; feeling pressurized to define herself in the terms of her partner. Such a situation creates little predictability and control over the resources at her disposal. In many cases depression, anxiety and other forms of mental distress may arise from an inability to confront the systems of dominance that are contributing to their difficulties. Indeed, women with independent economic resources have access to power and have been shown to suffer lower levels of depression.[55] Moreover, greater mental health is shown by women who have a greater degree of income parity with their husbands. When the structural roles of men and women are relatively similar, then the greater depression traditionally found in women no longer holds and the traditional gender divides in depression actually reverse in households where wives are the higher earners and do no more household labour than their partners. Such results suggest that the structural roles of women within society and the opportunities and responsibilities associated with these roles play an important role in these sex differences in depression. Indeed, post-natal depression has been considered to result from the isolation and seclusion of the mother together with demands regarding the early resumption of income making activity. If the political and economic demands of globalization are prolonged then their effect on the mental health of women can be expected to continue to be disproportionate as they contribute to the structural power imbalances that already affect women's mental health.

Ethnicity and Depression

Just as structural disenfranchisement has affected the mental health of women, so structural differences with regard to race are important in the experience of depression. The experience of women and ethnic minorities calls into question the belief that basic social processes work in the same way for different groups of people. We have already noted the importance of poverty and the way it can relate to depression, and this may be particularly important when recent estimates suggest that in non-metropolitan areas of the US, nearly 50% of older black people and 24% of older native Americans live in poverty.[88] Furthermore, in 1999, the poverty rate for all black Americans and Hispanic Americans was considerably higher than that for white Americans. When we appreciate that black men and women are around three times as likely to be unemployed as whites and that the net worth of white families is around ten times that of black families,[89] one might expect that the relationship between poverty and depression be particularly marked for ethnic minorities.

Ethnic minorities are subject to many of the same forms of structural discrimination and disempowerment as women. These include biased hiring practices, the presence of the 'glass ceiling' to curb promotion prospects, general discrimination, welfare stigma, greater exposure to violence, crime, economic disadvantage, single parenthood, exposure to health hazards and limited access to health care. They experience greater exposure to social isolation and feelings of second class citizenry as well as sometimes having to cope with the pressures and difficulties of acculturation into a new country and culture.

Earlier work suggested that there were no ethnic differences in depression between minority participants and whites in western research. In two research projects undertaken in the US in the late 1970s and early 1980s, no differences in depression were found between white, Hispanic and black participants[189] and between black participants and white participants.[190] However, recent work tends to suggest otherwise.[158,191,192] Minority participants experienced more depressive symptoms and a marginally higher prevalence of depression than white participants and these effects were mediated by participants struggling to meet their basic needs.[191] In another study, African–Americans and Hispanics exhibited elevated rates of major depression relative to whites and these elevated levels of depression were largely associated with greater health burdens and a lack of health insurance.[192] Furthermore, after controlling for differences in socioeconomic status, African–American women reported more symptoms of distress and Latino women were significantly more depressed than other groups. These ethnic differences were not moderated by education or employment. Different methods and samples can produce considerable variance in findings but ethnic differences in distress and depression appear to be important.

As well as possible differences in mental health status, ethnic minorities are exposed to different practices and interactions with professionals within the health system. African–Americans are less likely to receive care for depression than white

Americans, and health providers are less likely to detect mental disorders in black and Latino patients as compared to white patients.[193,194] An interesting study on physicians whose patients had coronary artery disease showed that black patients were more likely to be judged as non-compliant, less intelligent and be more likely to engage in substance abuse than white patients, and doctors had less affiliation toward them (this was true even after sex, age, income and education were controlled for).[195] Since this was true after controlling for education one can rule out the judgments being correct. It seems that many doctors hold inappropriate stereotypes and these beliefs will be unlikely to aid the communication barriers between doctors and minority patients. Since physician's attitudes influence their behaviour in medical care and their treatment decisions, this could be important for minority patients who are suffering with depression. Minority patients may be less likely to volunteer information and be less compliant in treatment and consultation if they perceive a poor consultation alliance. Indeed, minority patients do show a diminished use of specialized mental health services.[196] Lower rates of antidepressants are recommended for minority patients, possibly as a result of a lack of recognition by clinicians or, indeed, patients. Since minority patients are less likely to use antidepressants due to fear of addiction, greater skepticism over their efficacy and a greater cultural mistrust about being used as guinea pigs, this contributes to the increased risk of depression in this group.[193,197]

Depression in Context: A Warning for the Future

Government approaches to mental health issues tend to move in cycles and these cycles are influenced by financial structures, social ideologies and the technology available at the time. For instance, in the US, managed care has been developed to reduce inpatient utilization by reducing admissions and lengths of stays.[198] The number of mental health beds in the US has declined from 560,000 to 77,000 since the mid-fifties and the number of private hospitals has tripled in the last 30 years.

The financial responsibility for mental health has shifted in recent years and the broad dispersion of the mentally ill in residential facilities has meant that they have become difficult to follow. However, private health programmes do not generally cover rehabilitative long term care and, on evaluation by the National Alliance on Mental Illness, all US behavioural health care companies failed to provide a sufficient service to their users.[198] Health insurance coverage for mental health has traditionally been more restrictive than for physical health complaints and the 47% decrease in the average length of stay for mental health patients in managed care is twice that for non-mental health patients and will likely be detrimental to people suffering from depression who may benefit from longer-term treatment.[184]

In recent years, the UK has spent a lower proportion of its GDP on health care than European partners like France, Germany and Italy, and the 'Care in the Community' scheme has resulted in thousands of people with mental health problems effectively being made homeless. In many cases no long-term effort is made to help those who leave hospital with housing, medication, job training and other necessities and so increasing the chance of further mental health problems. To compound these changes, we have experienced a growth in the language of consumption regarding public health services. Prominent in the recent health provision literature has been a system of rhetoric that has more in common with corporate finance than the ethics of healthcare and reflects the gradual commodification of public health care in the UK.

We know that the number of people in poverty in the UK increased from 5 million to over 14 million between 1979 and 1992. This has occurred as we have come to embrace enterprise culture. With the rise of Thatcher and Reagan and their neoliberal disciples, we witnessed a growth in a system of international economics whose agenda has affected almost every area of our lives. This change in political and economic consensus has brought about an increase in a number of factors known to be precipitators of mental illness, and depression in particular. These have included greater inequality and poverty, reduced occupational rights, an increase in deleterious work practices and temporary unemployment. We have witnessed an increase in stressful life events, greater social isolation and reduced support, increased generational transmission of mental health problems, a greater cumulative burden for women and ethnic minorities, and an increasing exposure to the difficulties associated with crime and health problems. We are experiencing increases in behavioural disturbance, the breakdown of families, urban crowding and reduced quality of public services that, in combination, are driving what some are calling the epidemic of depression.

The Employable Units

This neoliberal Anglo-American model of capitalism takes as its fundamental baseline the isolation of people as employable units and then operates to disable all regulations and social norms that challenge such a perspective. As touched upon in the previous chapter, its success is predicated on minimizing any elements of our social and occupational worlds that remotely interfere with productivity and wealth accumulation, and it does this at the expense of the quality of life of a growing number of citizens, not only in the US and the UK, but around the world. While one might imagine that the role of the government would be to protect their citizen's from insecurity, recent free market driven developments have depended on destroying any vestige of collective power that might work to protect the quality of life and mental health of its citizens.

A democratic society depends on an informed citizenry making political choices that protect their livelihood and quality of life, but this is clearly at odds with the current Anglo-American system of politics whose profit-driven social order has a single interest in representing people in terms of their economic contribution. As transnational corporations continue to have their preferences realized, political debate and institutions are marginalized. Downsizing and outsourcing are viewed as regrettable but necessary and appropriate vestiges of a world order where economic competition between corporations, states and countries is the fundamental driving force of modern society.

However, this system has consequences. You cannot continue to exert this pressure on a society without something giving and that something is the mental health and well-being of its citizens. This is exactly what we are seeing today, and will continue to see in the future, as long as we are subject to the economic and social pressures that breed humiliation, powerlessness, inequality and increasing hardship. Ignoring these mental health factors in pursuit of short-term, corporate efficiency will eventually lead to long term health costs. The WHO note that after a single episode of depression, the likelihood of another episode is 50%, after two episodes it increases to 70% and after three episodes this likelihood increases to 90%.[9] More people will be exposed to the recurrent ravages of clinical depression.

The Individual and Mental Health

Public health has had a tendency to neglect the influence of structural elements of socioeconomic variance on mental health, but changes in social and economic policies that reduce inequality will improve the mental health of the population.[144] Putting aside the issue of reverse causality that pervades discussions of mental health and inequality, the very fact that poverty and exclusion are associated with depression should raise greater concern than it has, both in academic and political spheres. It is not unusual to read in the medical literature that longitudinal studies are needed to support the contention that poverty causes common psychiatric disorders like depression. I disagree. There is already sufficient evidence available to prompt political action were there a will to do so, but such economic and political action has not been realized because the governments and the decision makers in the business world are not motivated to make difficult changes that will penalize a system from which they benefit.

There is a missing economy of well-being and quality of life that has fallen by the wayside as Anglo-American capitalism continues to bring greater advantage to fewer people. It is not in the interests of the powerful to consider political and economic perspectives when addressing depression; perspectives that would include such broad domains as local planning issues, government deregulation, the influence of the media, and advertising and consumerism. Rather, we find the popular focus on the 'individualized' elements of mental distress, all crucial, but nonetheless only part of the story. Globalization is an isolating force and one of the side effects of this isolation is to present the individual as the unit of mental distress and treatment for this distress. When we hear prominent public servants (and academics in the mental health field) talk of the growing problem of depression and mental health, they often do so as if it represents some impenetrable mystery, insolvable by some of the greatest minds. This is because depression is a political and economic problem and one which does not always fit into the narrow discourses that are characteristic of individual disciplines. It is a problem relevant to the situations that people face in their day to day lives, situations that are governed, influenced and manipulated by others.

The European Commission Health and Consumer Protection Directorate General's recent 'Actions against depression' report notes that there are 'actions that can be taken at member, state, regional and local levels to reduce the impact of depression across Europe'.[1] The actions of the European Commission are legally based on Article 152 of the treaty, which dictates that a high level of human health protection shall be ensured in the definition and implementation of all community actions and policies, and yet the document above represents much of what is wrong with political approaches to mental health. It focuses on individual interventions and health care services with no appreciation of the macroscopic political context. Effective mental health policy requires a commitment to wider goals within society.

A political system has developed that means we are facing a genuine threat of significant increases in mental health problems and many involved in the mental health industry have been, if not complicit, then painfully ignorant in their promulgation of individual solutions. The mental health sciences can generally be characterized by the modernist and artificially polarized debate between the environment and the individual, as if the two exist in isolation. Even when the environment is focused on, it tends to be with an individual focus as we encounter discussion of the individual's environment and fails to focus on aspects of the environment that are not under individual control. We often behave as though environmental elements like life stress, financial strain, problems at work and gender are where the analysis should end. In actual fact they are where the analysis should begin as we try to understand the political and structural factors that perpetuate these elements.

Durkheim noted that 'every time a social phenomenon is explained by a psychological phenomenon we may be sure that the explanation is false'[124] and he was right. The mental health sciences and organized psychology have been achingly slow to even consider such a debate. A focus on the individual has only been partially effective, and usually complicitly ineffective, at addressing social questions and depression is now, more than ever, a social question. In the next chapter I discuss the way the mental health sciences, and psychology in particular, have played their part in this complicit ineffectiveness and are still contributing directly and indirectly to Anglo-American capitalism's manifestation of isolated units of employment.

Chapter 6
The Mental Health Sciences and the Depression Industry

To understand the way that psychotherapy and the mental health movement have developed over recent decades one has to travel back in time to the era(s) when the 'mind sciences' began to gain prominence in public and scientific discourses. The actual term 'psychotherapy' arose sometime towards the end of the nineteenth century but its origins go back to Greek antiquity. In ancient Greece and Rome, the cause and cure of many diseases was considered to result from supernatural or religious forces. A variety of cures were effected to address such diseases and they tended to range from incantations, charms and spells to people sleeping within the precincts of the local temple in order that God could counsel them in their dreams.

One of the first thinkers on record to address the importance of the spoken word as a cure was Gorgias (483–376 BC), who noted that the persuasive word acted upon the soul in an analogous fashion to the action of medicines upon the body. Words, even without the addition of magical power, could banish pain, remove fear and inspire compassion and happiness.[22]

Plato redefined mental illness and distress as elements of ignorance related to the excessive power of the appetite over the rational, a power that would lead inexorably to madness and vice. It was Plato who envisioned the philosopher as the physician of the soul, the man charged with helping to put man in touch with his 'true self'. Only then would he achieve what he called 'sophrosyne', moral sanity and a healthy soul. Through the musings of such philosophers as Cicero (106–43 BC) and Seneca (4 BC–65 AD), various troubling conditions came to be considered as disorders and the benefit of a good friend was recommended as a general panacea for mental disorders. A good friend was able to provide conversation that could soothe anxiety and assist in decision making. Galen (AD 129–200) also advised the benefits of counsel and guidance in the form of old, wise noblemen who had lived an excellent life and he believed that people could be cured by nothing more than such good counsel and persuasion.

Gradually, a change occurred where the magico-religious understanding of mental distress waned and patients were exposed to the healing power of words. New methods of faith healing grew from the practices and principles originally ascribed to Christianity.[199] Where Christianity had previously used counsel and penance to remedy sinful behaviour, the reformation created a problem with regard to the control of wicked and deviant behaviour since confession and penance was now voluntary.

When Mesmer's work grew in prominence in the eighteenth century, it represented for some the medicalization of a type of therapy that had previously belonged to the realm of the religion. Coleridge was not alone in his conjecture that the treatment of mental disease was best addressed by the physician who inspires hope. Magnetic rapport, although controversial, had been popularized by Mesmer and had contributed to the growing sympathy towards the concept of the listening healer.[8]

Chapter 2 gave an account of the way that the mental health sciences grew to find a role in a Victorian society. With the authority of the church under pressure from empiricist philosophers like Descartes, the material world was coming to be understood in terms devoid of religion and God. The rigorous maxims of science were resolved as the only way to truly understand the material world and the only way from civilization to enlightenment. With this contention, power moved from the church and the monarchy to secular institutions. The brutality of the mental health system was co-opted by the medical firmament and by the middle of Victoria's reign the medical profession had assumed control of representations of mental illness. With this came control of the asylums that had been used to restrain, imprison and torture many of the unfortunates who were unable to conform to the rules of society.

Cell theory, and the associated technologies, exploded at the end of the nineteenth century, with a concomitant objectification of medical patients. A focus on looking at rather than listening to was exemplified by the popularity of physiognomy and phrenology and a space opened up for a more person-centred, psychologically based therapy. Toward the end of this century, words were becoming the essential form of mental treatment and Freud and Breuer developed their concepts of psychodynamic theory. A patient's talk would eventually allow access to traumatic experience via hidden memories and these memories could be brought into awareness through psychotherapy. The memory, and the deleterious effects that were associated with the memory, could then be dissipated through the relationship between the therapist and the patient. Personality traits and psychological symptoms grew as the medical establishment created a context for understanding the psychology of the individual. The development of the 'self' and the popularity of the individualist ethic are covered in Chapter 2 and so we will take up psychology's story in the twentieth century.

One of the principle themes that arose at the end of the nineteenth century had been that sociopolitical problems be considered in psychological terms. The proponents of the positive thinking and mesmerist movements had come to provide the popular 'cure' for such problems. Such a focus allowed the structural social elements of mental distress to remain untouched while providing a basis for the development of an embryonic mental health industry. The concept of personality came to replace the traditional Victorian concept of 'character' and individual dispositions were no longer steadfastly judged by moral or religious codes.[54] There was a psychological element to disorders like neurasthenia, hysteria and the 'vapors'. Now that these psychological disorders had been medicalized, they would need a new therapeutic ethos to address their treatment and, depending on the class and status of the person, return them to society cured of their unfortunate dispositions.

By the early decades of the twentieth century, such words as 'psyche' and 'mind' had made the transition from the medical establishment to the popular vernacular and the spread of psychology and the mental health movement as the vehicle for remedying the psychological disorders of the populous was growing. The development of neurophysiology meant that mental disorders could be realized in terms of specific parts of the brain rather than the mind as a whole. In doing so this gave further credence to the localization of the origins of mental distress within the individual.

Psychoanalysis and other psychological treatments came to perfectly compliment the growing consumerism that people were experiencing. Freudian psychoanalysis was moving from the medical discourse into other discourses like deviance, personal problems and unhappiness. The workplace was an area where the intervention of psychological therapy allowed a platform for management to change legitimate complaints or difficulties experienced by workers into psychological symptoms. As discussed in Chapter 2, dynamic therapy linked disordered behaviour and normal behaviour as variants of common processes so that therapists could potentially treat anyone. It helped to occasion the turn inward in search of solutions to problems, away from the political and economic conditions that governed people's lives. One of the reasons that psychoanalytic psychotherapy became so popular in the US was that it neatly dovetailed with the existing social ethos of the country. The movement rebelled against the repressive nature of society and emphasized the needs and the rights of the individual and in doing so created the framework for the future growth of other forms of psychological therapy. Any everyday problems that people were experiencing, regardless of their genesis, were party to solution by the two growing strands of self-help available in society, psychoanalysis and consumer products. The individual's growth and fulfillment was portrayed as remediable by the growing diet, cosmetic, electronic equipment and self-improvement industries.[54]

The institution of social psychology had arisen from the manifest changes brought about by the industrial revolution where large groups of people had been brought together. Experimental social psychology, from its earliest inceptions, was a discipline that was clearly motivated and dominated by the political and economic ethos of the time. People now existed in big groups but a number of experiments were formulated in order to show how the individual was more effective than the social group.[200] Social psychology came to be represented by the practice of abstracting behaviour from its context and providing an individual motive, a practice that meant that no broad changes in the fabric of society would be necessary to cope with any problems that this new enquiring science might find.

World War II provided the momentum for a reconceptualization of the importance of environmental stressors and their role in the precipitation of mental illness. It also provided a new focus on information processing. The cognitive psychology movement gained momentum in the 1950s in parallel with the growth in computer technology that had arisen from the Second World War.[201] Those who modeled cognition on computers in the footsteps of Turing perpetuated the myth that a pure, disinterested knowledge exists in the human brain, much as with electronic computers. Such an approach meant that the representation of knowledge was abstracted and removed from its social and political reference points and this simplistic ethos is still attractive for many who consider themselves cognitive scientists today.

One of the principle tenets of cognitivism was to reduce the 'different' to 'the same' using far-fetched electronic analogies where machines and humans came to be viewed in equivalence. This approach tended not to incorporate the possibility that human beings play an active part in selecting, attending and shaping their environment and that they themselves are shaped by powerful social and political forces that provide the basis for much of their knowledge. Indeed some embraced the reductionist elements of the cognitive approach with a zeal that would have shaken Darwin.

At around the same time dynamic society was beginning to fall out of favour and the early 1960s saw a growth in the application of scientific falsification.[55] As was discussed in earlier chapters, the nebulous nature of dynamic psychiatry meant that such an application of scientific principles would never operationalize. This, together with the increased financial accountability for mental health services and the growing protest movement and medical focus within the mental health industry led to a reduction in its popularity. The reasoning behind the move towards classification had little to do with clinical intuitions and more to do with economic imperatives. Western society needed a system of mental health classification (the DSM-III) that would respond to the economic challenges of the day and this primarily set the agenda for the definitions and conceptualizations of many mental illnesses that we currently embrace.

Through teaching and practice, the DSM system of categorization (and its European equivalent, the ICD-10) has come to be seen more and more as the natural order of a discrete psychiatry. Its genesis in terms of non-clinical imperatives has been, if not forgotten, then certainly marginalized in the stories of psychiatry and psychology, allowing both discourses to be represented as two of the last bastions of modernity. Even if such historical categorization was accepted unreservedly, the disparities that have been found between the two major psychiatric classifications systems[143] should prompt a healthy degree of skepticism. Indeed the discovery of certain culturally sanctioned disorders in recent years could also be considered to throw doubt on the validity and reliability of some of the categories that have been developed by the psychiatric firmament. Issues that were previously presented as normal events in the course of a woman's life have been represented as psychological disorders in recent years. Premenopausal dysphoric disorder, post-partum depression and perimenopausal depression are classic examples of the 'bracket creep' that is increasingly addressed with psychotropic medication.[202] I am not suggesting that such experiences do not exist, or in some way are not worthy of treatment, quite the contrary. What I would say is that perhaps such continued malleability in the categorizations over a relatively short period of time should introduce a degree of caution to our appraisal of their validity.

Those in defense of the changing nature of the mental health classification trends have noted that professionals and the public have become more aware of certain conditions and so recognition follows. But can such an explanation really account for the growing popularity of such conditions as social phobia, a disorder that did not officially exist before 1980 but that had reached an estimated prevalence of 13.3% in the US by the early 1990s?[55] The fact that we have witnessed a quadrupling of mental health professionals in the US between 1970 and 1995 and have bestowed increasing responsibility on mental health professionals to address crime, social disruption, deviance and bad habits has undoubtedly perpetuated such categorical flux. In 1994 in the state of California alone there were 13,800 clinical psychologists, 13,000 social workers, 21,600 marriage and family guidance counselors and 6,500 psychiatrists.[54] Indeed North America now has more therapists than firefighters and mail carriers and twice as many as dentists.[203] DSM-IV now classifies nearly 400 distinct mental disorders and configuring all of these disorders as natural entities rather than cultural constructions becomes more difficult when they come to cater for children who do not behave in class or who eat too much.

Substituting the Personal for the Political

The overwhelming focus on the individual is a particularly western way of thinking about people and the mental health problems that they experience. Such constructs are supported by those with the power to create public representations of the self, be it those in medicine, the media, politics or other domains where people have the power to define what it is to be human and what does and does not constitute a problem or a disease. Distress, suffering and mental disorder are very real parts of everyday life and if you work in the mental health sciences and the healing industry then you are automatically part of a powerful consensus that creates the boundaries of everyday living.

The mental health sciences today are no different from a number of other industries in that different factions defend their personal interests but such defenses are not always conducive to the best interests of patients and service users. Scientific psychology and psychiatry play a fundamental role in public mental health and both are still very much entrenched in a culture of modernism where tools are utilized in order to attain the unique truth that will lead to the 'cure' of a given disorder. Such a preoccupation with universal laws and universal truths has created an ideological agenda that has tended to move in synchrony with the political and economic ethos of the day. The impossibility of existing outside of cultural contexts has been resolutely downplayed by the psychological sciences as they have continued to plough their furrow in search of universal truths and universal selfhood. The local nature of time and place has been paid lip service with the local usually constructed as the straw man in simplistic polarized dyads like the individual versus society debate that is scrutinized in many universities today.

The process of classifying human behaviours, and the people who undertake such behaviours, will always be more beneficial for some than for others and such constructions cannot but be the product of ideology. The psychological sciences have privileged access to concepts of mental illness at present and this hegemony requires certain assumptions to be supported, one of which is that individual processes are the source of mental distress.

For as long as the psychological sciences fail to fully appreciate the structural causes of emotional difficulties that were discussed in Chapter 5, they perpetuate the power of these structural arrangements. Ahistorical theories appeal to a great many academics, not least because they have been schooled in, and propagated, such theories for a great many years. A sudden change to appreciating the locality and construction of knowledge, to appreciating the structural factors that create the perspectives that we use to understand suffering and an acceptance of multiple 'truths' is not a perspective that infuses easily into the traditional psychological sciences. Such an approach questions the medical authority under which these sciences have operated for many years. Mainstream mental health sciences represent the history of psychology as an apolitical discourse, removed from histories of oppression. While a small minority in the field challenge these representations, the tenets of scientific modernism still hold the fort and will continue to do so for the foreseeable future.

Traditional psychological sciences offer an individual location of power rather than political transformation, a state of affairs that have led prominent feminists to critique psychology as a 'pseudo-scientific buttress for patriarchal ideology and social organization'.[203] Personal explanations of mental health and mental disorder have been presented in the place of political explanations and this has tended to disguise the very real social and material disenfranchisement felt by large groups of people in society. The quest to seek individual solutions is the quest to continue to support this structural disenfranchisement and perpetuate sexism, racism, classism and pretty much any other 'ism'. Such a focus on the self-contained individual reifies the approach itself by magnifying the individual as the object of visibility. The more that the individual is focused on as the unit of scientific surveillance, the more it appears to be the 'correct' unit to come under scrutiny when seeking solutions to social problems. And if such an approach should coincide with the political and economic 'truth' of the time then even more powerful will it become.

Whilst one could present a case for the principles of chemistry and physics (although certainly not their applications) existing outside of political persuasion, the psychological sciences are never apolitical. Any discourse that has the power to construct psychological knowledge and impose a given set of definitions results in coercive practice at some level. Moreover the sanctioning of a given set of knowledge constructs provides a powerbase for the constructors of this knowledge. Indeed Foucault suggested that the very creation of the psychological sciences was based on a need to police the more deviant and unruly members of society.[200]

A straightforward application of the principles of scientific testability, without consideration of who is doing the scientific testing and why they are doing it, is dangerously naïve, certainly so for whoever stands to lose out as a result of the findings that such scientific practice uncovers. The ideologies that we embrace in the psychological sciences provide the framework not just for scientific ideas but for the continuation of the hegemonic power and material gains experienced by those external forces that support, produce and disseminate such ideologies. The modern psychological sciences, with their focus on individualizing personal and social problems, have, as one might expect, received grand support from the far and centre right (which, in the current political climate, is almost everyone) as such explanations remove structural culpability from the political realm.

Concepts of power are represented by the psychological sciences in such a way that personal power has become interchangeable with group or political power.[58] Power is the capacity that people have to control or influence the terms on which their daily lives operate. Treatment, research and teaching in the psychological sciences are often part of the process of disempowerment as they ignore structural power inequalities. More than that, defining power and 'feeling empowered' in personal terms allows the creation of such concepts as 'inner power', which are used to replace and denigrate concepts of group power. However, this creation of sources of power solely attributed to the individual person is a substandard replacement for political and economic power. Working to bring a feeling of personal inner power to single mothers who are working two or three jobs on top of childcare is unlikely to substantiate a significant change in their social and economic circumstances. Power in the arena of public policy is required to change structural relations that make many people's lives so difficult. A prominent focus on self-empowerment, self-discovery and self-validation leads to the belief that independence equals empowerment but in reality this could not be further from the truth.

Psychology's Artificial Dichotomies: The Individual Versus Society Argument

Over the years, those involved in the psychological sciences have become adept at creating and then reifying theoretical dichotomies that fail to withstand even the gentlest scrutiny. Many of the terms used in these discourses operate to prevent alternative considerations.[79] They set the terms within which a debate occurs. For instance, the speculation focused on the redundant individual versus society argument, which is still alive and well in contemporary psychology teaching, is the perfect example of such an institutionalized and pervasive tactic. Through such debates the psychological sciences work to separate the individual and society with the result that students understand individuals as torn from the cultural and political contexts upon which they are then subject to various theoretical conjecture and different types of experimentation. Such an approach supports prominent individualist political discourses as well as providing a convenient research context for the discipline. It is considerably harder to undertake scientific investigations on the ways in which people interact with the structural components of their political and economic environment. Or indeed the ways that such structures lead to limiting or beneficial circumstances within which their quality of life can be defined.

Many of the concepts employed within the psychological sciences are independent of proper social behaviour[204] but these concepts, once formalized, gather momentum as research and clinical careers start to form around them.[55] Furthermore, and especially in the realm of mental illness, the abstraction of the psychological individual has provided a context for lay advocacy groups who are motivated by the presentation of biological rationales for many mental illnesses. Powerful groups like the National Alliance for the Mentally Ill (NAMI), with influence in the US congress, are working to reduce the stigma associated with mental illness by deemphasizing such theory as faulty parenting styles and oedipal conflicts and focusing on the importance of biology. While such biological perspectives are undoubtedly crucial in our greater understanding of mental illness, such a dominant focus on individual factors belies the fact that there are structural, economic and social conditions, especially under the current context of globalization, that play a role in the suffering of the mentally ill and their families. To exclude these in a stigma-reduction exercise may be counter-productive.

The Identification of Separation: Modernity, Progress and Common Sense

The modern era that followed the enlightenment placed the assumption of continual progress and universality of application at the forefront of intellectual inquiry. Irrationality was to be replaced with reason and empirically validated knowledge was to replace superstition. Science was the tool of this progress, the means by which universal laws and regulations could be uncovered and such an approach has been important in providing the framework for the classification ethos. Nature was considered to be lawful and science would discover the laws. Such a view, however, fails to capture the nature of human experience and behavioural disturbances. The same kinds of behaviours can have very different underlying problems and two people with a similar mental health problem such as depression can experience this in very different ways. Universality in the behavioural sciences is still a guiding principle even though scientific action is embedded in culture and in values and systems with political and economic rules.

This commitment to progress in the psychological sciences has seen the automatic repudiation of approaches that do not use similar methods of enquiry as somehow inferior and untrustworthy.[205] It has also led to an obsession with being modern. Despite two world wars, the development of atomic weapons and the holocaust,[206] the remnants of the modernist tenet of progress has emphasized a focus on the recent and the modern as work from the past is often sidelined as irrelevant. As a result much interesting work falls by the wayside as we automatically assume that current work supersedes that of the past. Such a focus allows the psychological sciences to protect and distance themselves from some of the more questionable concepts that have been popular and definitive in its recent past (i.e. the pathology of homosexuality).

The psychological sciences not only have a need to be distanced from their own questionable past but also from lay theories of human behaviour. To be effectively organized as a discipline requires that the discipline can provide a service not available from outside of the discipline. The psychological sciences are constantly under pressure to prove their knowledge as separate from common knowledge and creating the distinction between what lay people know about human behaviour and what the psychological sciences know has received a great deal of focus within the discipline.[200] A brief glance at some of the prominent literature within psychology will highlight a discipline that is formulated to transcend the naivety of common sense but such discursive labour arouses as much suspicion as it seeks to quell.

Scientism and the Distrust of Concepts of Morality

The American Psychological Association (APA) has stated that promoting human welfare is one of its primary roles.[207] Forgetting for a minute psychology's history in the arena of social management and control, to take such an aim at face value is to accept fundamentally the tenets of universality and progress. By focusing on the individual as the unit of analysis, the psychological sciences are promoting some human's welfare, some of the time, and manifestly denigrating that of others. Individualization demands the removal of the structural context and with it goes the capacity to effect change at a level beyond the person. The psychological sciences' recent history of improving human welfare is hardly a ringing endorsement of their benevolent intentions. In the UK in the 1970s, there was an 'illness' known as 'state benefit neurosis', which involved the disorder of refusing to take a lowly paid job when more money was available through the benefits of the state.[203] Going further back, 'drapetomania' was a disease suffered by slaves when they were apt to try to flee from the often brutal tendencies of their masters on the US slave plantations. The classification labels used by the psychological sciences have not always worked in the interests of promoting human welfare.

The theories of the psychological sciences do not always arise out of the process of objective scientific inquiry, rather the cultural context within which such inquiries are embedded. This is true of behavioural disturbances and the way that we conceptualize such disturbances depends less on scientific theory and more on cultural norms. Society generates concepts and the data and theories tend to follow.[206] When the APA removed homosexuality from the category of pathological disorders, this was not due to ground-breaking research findings that provided evidence for its sudden shift to 'normality', rather it was due to a change in the social climate and organized protest.

The pseudoscientific nature of many of the practices of the psychological sciences is generally well disposed towards attack from within the discipline but not the discipline itself. Attacking the quality of a piece of research is acceptable since such an attack can be represented, and refuted, in the context of positivism; attacking the actual structure of the discipline and the practices that it sanctions and legitimizes is unacceptable and is likely to result in professional exclusion from constructive debate.

So how does this relate to the mission statement regarding human welfare? It is fundamentally important because even if we ignore the historical precepts above and accept the human welfare mission as a coherent and trouble-free concept, we arrive at one of the great ironies that trouble the psychological sciences. To allow any concept of human welfare to dominate the practices of your discipline is a funda-mentally moralistic act. The desire to work toward, and use science to achieve, an increase in human welfare is not a scientific act but an act that seeks to follow the principles of 'right conduct'. As such it belongs in the ethical and moral domain. This itself is not such a problem unless we look closer at the treatment of morality within the discipline. That is because the psychological sciences fundamentally mistrust the concept of morality.

The mainstream psychological sciences have been constructed as being governed by objective, value-free practices but as we saw earlier with homosexuality, this is clearly not the case. The moral agenda is considered to be irrelevant to the construction of knowledge by science. It has no place within a discipline where scientific medical enquiry supports randomized controlled trials that produce results based on rational and testable hypotheses. However, the psychological sciences are involved in decisions as to what is right and wrong and what is appropriate and inappropriate and the DSM-IV classification is infused with ideas of appropriate and inappropriate behaviour. Personal and social value is fundamental to the classification systems adhered to and the brand of morality that is perpetuated happens to be white, middle-class, liberal capitalist and predicated around individual problems and solutions.

One might be justifiably wary of multinational industries that purport to work towards the betterment of human welfare and then use value-free scientific discourse to achieve those ends. This has particular implications for the construction of psychological therapies for those with mental health problems.

Psychotherapy and Isolation: Promoting the Self (Part 1)

We currently have an economy that fervently promotes consumer ideology. It is a consumer ideology that works in perfect harmony with a mental health industry that treats the unfortunate mental health effects of such consumerist rhetoric. For as long as the mental health industry is conceived of within a framework that speaks the language of individualism and self-hood, and minimizes the importance of political and economic forces, such an industry will continue to contribute to the problems that it has been charged with healing.

The therapy industry is one of the primary standards of western mental health. However, as well as effectively treating mental health problems for many people, it can also contribute to these problems in a number of ways. Its general focus on the individual self and individual dispositional characteristics as the site(s) of action for common mental health problems like depression serves to marginalize the political, economic and structural systems that leave people and groups in society in positions that increase their likelihood of experiencing mental distress.

Regardless of the rhetoric of conservatives and the radical and centre right, isolation from the family and social structures is the most effective way to mobilize an efficient workforce in the twenty-first century. Social groups, social ties, families and any other connections that contribute to social capital and collective power, and that may bring inertia to the neoliberal project, are simply expendable. This is one of the reasons why the therapy industry dovetails so well with the contemporary political and economic imperatives. We have a psychological treatment that complements, and has grown to meet the needs of, the current political ethos.

This isolation complements the cultural imperative of creating and maintaining isolated economic units with little recourse to the structural and democratic support with which to improve quality of life, employment rights and work towards regulations that will halt the continual growth in inequality. What is more, having played a role in working towards this construction of people in terms of economic units, psychotherapy is charged with the treatment of the mental problems that have arisen as a result of this construction. We have a positive feedback loop where psychotherapy helps to build the structure of western society and then addresses the problems that arise from this construction. The mentally disenfranchised, those that find it difficult to adapt and flourish as societies' safety nets fall by the wayside, are told that they cannot be helped by those around them, that only the techniques, procedures and expertize of the therapy industry can address their desperation.

And then we have the almost perversely entertaining irony that academic psychology and academic psychiatry secure research funds in the quest to understand the stigma and the causes of mental illness. This, despite constructing a framework that excludes political and structural culpability, and hence reducing mental distress to the level of the individual. So what are the results of this reduction? Perhaps not surprisingly the consensus grows that people are to blame for their own mental distress. They must be if they are the unit of treatment for this distress. After all a therapy session with a single mother who is suffering from the most debilitating depression does not treat the advertizers who create a constant need for her children to have the new consumer accoutrements or the government and corporate decision makers for reducing her probability of receiving a good education or trapping her in consistent and growing poverty and helplessness. They do not treat a succession of governments that contributed to the erosion of her employment rights, that have contributed to her reduced job security and poor pay; that means she can spend less time with her children and family and friends. They do not treat the media who create a perception of single mothers as welfare scroungers. So whose fault must it be that they are on the verge of breakdown? It must be the individual's fault. Noone is denying that people make bad choices, that they can play a part in the decisions that lead to difficulties in their lives and that they can fail to take responsibility for decisions that can lead towards their own distress. However, removing the importance of the structural framework within which we live is a dangerous misrepresentation.

The bad things that we experience on a day-to-day basis have been removed from our communities and social environments into therapy where individuality, self-reliance and self-fulfillment are emphasized as positive life choices (as opposed to a reliance or dependence on structures and people outside of the self). Psychotherapy highlights the importance of finding the 'real self' and the 'true self', as if many choices up until now had been made by a false self shackled to the chains of societies and communities on which they depend and are inevitably let down. Only the independent client, when creating an atmosphere of self-reliance, can come to terms with, and address, the problems that affect them on a day-to-day basis. This process of supposed empowerment is very much a form of compensation for the structural inequalities under which they labour and to which real, meaningful power is related. There is no self without context and to assume this is hopelessly simplistic. We know ourselves though the institutions that shape us; our communities, our jobs, our families and friendships, and solutions that separate us from this context are separating us from institutionalized sources of difficulties.

I am not suggesting a conspiracy of psychological therapists who meet regularly to think of ways that they can support the neoliberal agenda and generate as much suffering as they can possibly treat. The vast majority of therapists are decent, kind people whose intuition is to help those in distress. What I am saying is that the current system of psychotherapy has evolved to compliment the economic, political and media consensus as well as to indirectly provide support for its own discourses by individualizing mental distress and treating the effects of structural difficulties. The Anglo-American ethos of personal responsibility for every experience in our lives, good and bad, is far removed from our social reality. If you do not have money or love or peace then it is your fault. You are the complete agent of responsibility in this capitalist fantasy.

Commodifying the Skilled Helper

The focus on the individual as the site of inquiry and action, and the therapeutic relationship as the source of individual healing, works to increase the isolation and decrease the social capital that a person will experience. We have reached the point where, in partially serving the need to carve out a professional industry, only professional therapists have been conceptualized as being able to provide the comfort and healing necessary for people suffering with mental health problems, and specifically, depression. The continual redefining of problems as psychiatric and individual in nature, and requiring intervention that can only be provided by an expert therapist, can work to limit the extent to which people feel that they can reach out to one another and to use the support and strength of friends and family. Thus, the isolationism that pervades twenty-first century western society is implicitly encouraged by the incredible growth of the therapy industry and its self-imposed standards of professional practice.

The growth and medical validation of the therapy industry over the last 40 or so years has led to a culture where people worry that they are treading where only qualified therapeutic experts should be treading. The therapist is an objective and empathic cipher, immune to possible abuses of power, judgments and assumptions. Medical validation has allowed the establishment of the therapy industry as a financially viable entity that provides a specialist service not available to others without training. Such an outlook can be dangerous as it disempowers 'normal' people from the context of being a 'helper' and reduces their involvement in the common mental disorders of their friends and families. Such disempowerment reduces one of the fundamental elements of community and friendship and contributes to a degree of isolation between those who are struggling and those who want to help but do not believe themselves qualified to do so. An element of the 'social being' is removed from the community and placed in the hands of a qualified stranger either for money or through the strictures of the medical estab-lishment. Being able to listen and to communicate are constructed as specialist skills that need to be taught and here lies the justification for the psychotherapeutic practitioner, trained in these very skills and how to apply them to those who are mentally distressed.

One of the results of the growth in this industry is the commodification of empathy and listening. Like all industries, the psychotherapy industry has competitors that have to be marginalized and these competitors can take the form of normal human relations and friendships. We now have a financed pseudo-simulation of companionship that, although undoubtedly very useful for some, can be considered to be replacing social institutions whose removal may be the partial or complete cause of the problem in the first place.

The Positive Business of Psychotherapy

Psychotherapy exists as a part of the problem that supports and constrains the dispositional representation of political issues but for many people it is also the solution. This is a paradox, not borne out of any intentional grand design but a side effect of a political and economic system that inevitably rewards individualist discourses. That psychotherapy is charged with providing the cures to the ills of society is somewhat perverse and has meant that therapy as a business is booming. To make people mentally distressed is not the intention of mental health professionals but many are complicit in a greater system whose effects are exactly that. That they profit from picking up the pieces is an effect of such a system.

The last 30 years have seen a profound growth in the neoliberal political consensus and this project has been served by both public and private forms of therapeutic practice. With private psychotherapy, the therapist is the agent only of the patient, whereas in public health care, the therapist is the agent of the institution that provides the service.[199] In the case of the UK National Health Service, this is the state. The individualist focus is dominant in both contexts since it facilitates the continued pop-ularity of private psychotherapy and facilitates the political and social agenda of the state in public service. In a centre right state under growing neoliberal influence, this is to ensure that people are productive and financially motivated consumers. The agenda of the state is to bring an individual back into work. We are in an era where UK employment advisors create solutions by offering General Practitioners financial incentives to force people on benefits back to work. Under plans unveiled recently, employment advisors are to be stationed in GP's surgeries to make it more difficult for doctors to sign people off.[208] This attempt to make doctors policemen for the Department for Work and Pensions is a very conscious and deliberate manipulation of the mental health system for political benefit. It is easy to understand the success of a state-sanctioned psychological treatment that addresses political factors in terms of personal pathologies.

However, I do not believe that therapists are motivated by the prospect of promoting a culture of isolation, one that fulfils the ideological criteria of modern capitalism. I suspect that they enter the discipline because they want to help people who need help and in many cases they do.

Despite the somewhat cynical perspective presented thus far, the story of psychotherapy is not as straightforward as a good guy/bad guy scenario. Psychotherapy is an industry that is often the last refuge for the truly desperate and bereft. Psychotherapists have the responsibility of addressing some of the most desperate people in society, a situation which in itself has profound political ramifications. They are responsible for guiding people as they make sense of their world, of themselves and of their problems. On the one hand, its damage can be insidious and pervasive. However not everyone has the social and community resources available to support them in their time of need. Or indeed not everyone wants to access these resources as a result of the stigma associated with societal conceptions of mental health problems and their economic relevance. Psychotherapy, whilst contributing to the personalizing of political sources of distress and pain, can also provide people with a great source of comfort. To deny this would be to oversimplify the argument and negate the experience of a great many people who have found effective solace in the support and guidance of a warm and empathic therapist.

As a means of communicating distress when a person may have no other avenues of expression, it can be very useful for some people with depression. Discomfort, pain and an inability to function as they want to and need to leads to a desire to address aspects of the person's life that they may not be able to address themselves. Many of psychotherapy's most vociferous critics like Celia Kitzinger and Rachel Perkins[203] point out the importance of utilizing social support to help people through depression and, while this is undoubtedly true, not everyone has that facility. Furthermore, there are therapists working outside the traditional schools who take a systemic approach that places a greater emphasis on the structure of social systems when contextualizing distress.

However, although psychotherapist's attempts to 'empower' their patients may well be assisting them in increasing a sense of control, they often remain firmly situated within an oppressive social context. Hence it can give a partial but illusory sense of agency in their world.[58] There are two levels of acquisition, that of power personally and of power in society. Therapy can often help one but diminish the other and hence actually work to diminish both forms of power.

Therapy as the Solution for Depression

Lord Layard, the UK government's 'happiness tsar', recently called for an extra 10,000 therapists to provide help for the record number of people whose lives are blighted by depression.[209] Layard blamed National Health Service cutbacks for the inability of many people to be able to access treatment. While one can follow his logic, this feels like blaming a lack of synthetic insulin for the many people suffering from diabetes. Perhaps Lord Layard and his happiness professionals could be focusing on the underlying causes of the increase in depression in the UK rather than focusing solely on the lack of treatments.

In any case, therapy is often not useful or appropriate for people with different types of clinical depression and is not recommended as a first port of call for treatment.[9] To represent psychotherapy, or a given type of psychotherapy, as the solution for all people with depression is a fallacy. It can address dysfunctional thoughts but in many cases these are symptoms rather than causes of the illness. What it usually cannot do is change their poverty, life stresses, financial strain, rising local crime, gender discrimination, occupational problems and exposure to the culture of commodification that have contributed to their psychological distress. Therapy will not cure depression in a great many cases. It can provide feelings of subjective comfort and can be effective for people whose depression may be very acutely associated with a given set of mutable circumstances but for many it is simply a source of empathy and support, useful in itself but not addressing the long-term socioeconomic precursors.

Depression is a biological, emotional and psychological illness that simply cannot be addressed with therapeutic exercises like thought monitoring. Some believe that a cognitive appraisal of one's world is primary in depression[10] but even if this was so it does not automatically mean that depression can be solved by addressing cognitive errors, that the process can be reversed through the same mechanisms. I believe that the full emotional, cognitive and physiological expression of the illness is beyond such an approach. Moreover it has been suggested that there is very little difference in efficacy between the different types of psychotherapies; the relationships between the client and the practitioner is the crux of any success achieved by clients.[55] A compassionate and empathic attitude is key.

A Celebration of the Interior

Anyone who has been exposed to any number of US made-for-television movies will be aware of the particularly individualist dogma encapsulated in the phrases 'listening to your heart' or 'following your dreams'. Such concepts seem to rely on the intuition that inside us resides a special place, untouched by the ravages of society; a place that we are free to access, that will direct us to the true path of righteousness, a path that has been debased and warped by the realities of our social worlds. Our personal experience can barely be trusted as we have been exposed to this perverse exterior dystopia and only inside, at the heart of the 'self', do we find the purity to guide us through the dark times towards our goal.

Such ideas as this are pervasive in the entertainment to which we are exposed. They are based on capitalist mantras that emphasize a disembodied sense of wellbeing and a distrust of the process of thinking about our exterior existence. Moreover, they have been supported by the more scientific ruminations of the psychological sciences. In many cases, psychotherapy subjugates political and intellec tual thought, replacing it with more conservative concepts of 'instinct' or 'feeling', concepts that exist outside of justification, no matter that they may exist as platitudes and meaningless aphorisms. This becomes a celebration of the 'hippie ethic', a nostalgic and conservative school of thought that places an unwarranted premium on what is 'natural' and 'instinctive'. In doing so it promotes self interest and a general lack of regard for our responsibilities to others in our community.

One of the principal points to note during the teaching of many psychotherapy courses is that no one is ever wrong. There is no such thing as subjective value judgments, no political or moral exigencies. There is little recognition of the political importance of taking an utterly non-judgmental attitude to teaching therapists. This approach strips political implications from actions so that we are left with platitudes that enable movement through the training process. It also means that our new fleet of counselors also adopts an apolitical stance. How does this wholesale rejection of political meaning influence the discipline? It means that there is no right or wrong. Societal issues are left untouched, while clients are encouraged to retreat into their interiors. Individuation is the haven for those encountering interactions that they find unfavourable and social issues remain relatively unscathed whilst the client gains a personal sense of wellness.

Whose Knowledge Is Created in Therapy?

The construction of meaning is intimately tied to issues of power. However, current practice in psychotherapy tends to neglect this maxim and institutionally minimizes the relationship between the knowledge 'created' by the therapeutic dyad and the power balance inherent in the relationship. However, any mutual knowledge concerning the life circumstances of the client will be closely related to issues of power concerning the therapist and the client and between their belief systems. The process often involves the supplanting of one social and political belief system with that of another with inevitable financial implications. Therapy induces the value system congruent to the therapist, which is usually a middle-class liberal-humanist set of values. Systems of oppression and social inequality are downplayed such that all clients from all places have access to the same validation for their distress. Everyone is equal in the eyes of the law and their therapist.

But, of course everyone is not equal. Some people and some groups are severely disadvantaged as a result of factors outside of their control and their therapist's control. That is not to say that people from certain structural backgrounds have greater validity to their distress, just that the psychotherapy industry has institutionally downplayed structural causes in the mistaken belief that this is necessary to validate individual distress. It is possible to appreciate the validity of individual distress without conceptualizing clients as being equal in social and political terms. But psychotherapy is largely a middle-class endeavour and such endeavours substantiate a status quo that works to the (comparative) benefit of those within that class, a class that exists regardless of Tony Blair's disingenuous assertion that we finally live in a classless society.

In the UK, the whole process of training as a therapist to chartered status costs several thousand pounds (post-degree) and this contributes to making the occupation amenable to prospective trainees with financial means. One of the results of this is that we have an emphasis on class-specific language and ideas that serve to remove the experience of therapists from the experience of some of their clients. Those who concur with their therapist's politics are often defined as mature and 'self actualized' whilst those who do not are rejected as lacking insight or 'resistant'. Psychotherapy is a consumer service and the meanings created by this service are political constructions that displace or subvert other constructions of misery, distress and despair. These constructions have a profound impact at the societal level. Certain narrative possibilities are encouraged and exemplified if they fall within a solution-focused individualistic rubric but should this not be the case then they can be disabled or neglected as counter-productive or without use. The practices that are supported within therapeutic relationships provide a context for understanding distress that supports specific forms of power at the cost of negating other constructions of power.

Regardless of what is preached by the therapy industry, qualities such as insightfulness, empathy, warmth and genuineness are qualities that can only be taught to a certain degree. The psychotherapy industry perpetuates its institutionalization by teaching that anyone can be a therapist and, indeed, a good therapist, by following a given set of training tenets. To do otherwise would remove the applicability of a number of potential future therapists and their tuition fees. This is why therapists are almost always described as 'experienced' rather than 'good'. Experienced suggests an accumulation of knowledge that is available just by being a part of the discipline for a given period of time, whereas good suggests an inherent ability that could be separate from time spent within the discipline. The concept of good is dangerous to the institutionalized structure of psychotherapy and so is often missing from the discourse. I have little doubt that, with guidance, almost anyone can improve on the above tenets but some therapists will always be better or more effective than others because they are able to provide these qualities as a result of a number of factors outside of industry training.

In the UK, in order to combat the huge increase in the number of people who suffer from depression and other common mental disorders, recent work has seen the introduction of computerized counseling programmes like 'Beating the Blues' and 'Fearfighter' as a cost-effective solution to this increase in National Health Service resources. Indeed in 2006, Beating the Blues, a programme that uses the tenets of cognitive behavioural therapy, is to be used in four East Sussex Primary Care Trusts for patients with mild or moderate depression by way of acting as a 'virtual therapist'. This is an example of the psychological sciences displaying such isolationist tendencies that contact with another human being is no longer seen as necessary. One wonders if such approaches might further contribute to the experience of disconnection that so many people feel, especially those with common mental disorders.

Psychology as Entertainment

It would not be quite right to leave this section on the psychological sciences and mental health without giving mention to the recent growth in the use of television psychologists and psychiatrists. The culture of symbiosis between the psychological sciences and modern consumerism has been more overtly expressed with the growth of media psychologists in recent years. Taking advantage of perceptions of the limited mental health literacy of the general public, as well as their own hard won status as experts in the behaviour of human beings, some psychologists (admittedly a select group) have come to inhabit a space in the enormously popular culture of reality television where their status as prophets of the obvious appears to be irrelevant to their popularity with media executives. These professionals use their clinical experience to extol the psychological virtues and limitations of a number of contestants for the entertainment of a mass audience. Their success appears to be based upon making reflections similar to those made by normal viewers but using language that is riddled with psychological jargon in order to suffuse an air of authority.

The benevolent aspect of the psychological sciences is represented by the culture of psychotherapy and the concomitant ethical implications of respecting the patient and striving to most effectively address their clinical needs. Unfortunately ethical considerations are far from paramount when some psychologists undertake work on the television. Their job is to describe, and hence contribute to, the formation of distress for mass entertainment with no compunction to help the people in distress. Such behaviour is usually justified on the basis that the reality contestants have chosen to enter into these distressing situations and can withdraw at any time. Or that, perversely, the mental health professionals are bringing the benefits of psychology as a discipline to a wider audience (although I struggle to see the benefits of representing your discipline by humiliating disadvantaged, distressed and usually working class or underclass contestants who have been removed from their usual cultural points of reference).

Television psychologists are usually confident enough to give descriptions and prescriptions without knowing anything at all about the background and life history of the subjects on which they comment. Curiously, these reflections on contestant's self-esteem, self-image and other self constructs emerge without any acknowledgement that much of their behaviour is the result of being placed in an artificial environment where so much of their context is manipulated by others (usually television producers) and under conditions of enormous stress. And yet the pathological behaviour or negative reactions that they exhibit are often construed as resulting from characteristics of the individual. God forbid that these incredibly stressful, artificial and vulnerable environments might play a part.

Media psychologists interact with the mental health story much like a journalist might in that they need to present it in the context of entertainment. As such, mentally curious, unbalanced or unpopular people are deconstructed by television doctors for the publics' entertainment. This does not improve the levels of stigma associated with mental health issues, indeed the very opposite. I suspect that most of these television mental health experts and psychologists would say they are doing no wrong but this is self-denial of epic proportions. Indeed one might suggest that many of these 'experts' crave celebrity in just the same way that their subjects do, only many hide behind their badges of medicine, authority and objectivity. The rise of media psychologists, and their incursions into magazines, news and current affairs programmes, has been swift. However, their 'clinical' analyses of contestant behaviours have contributed to the denigration of their own disciplines and, when they are complicit in the creation of psychological distress, the fundamental human rights of their 'victims'.

Medication and the Drug Industry: Promoting the Self (Part 2)

The theoretical rationale for the use of medicinal substances to benefit physical and psychosocial ailments has its roots in Hippocrates and Galen's humoral theories of illness and the need to strive for balance is still profoundly influential in many forms of medicine and the health supplement industry. The emergence of bacteriology and the discovery of microorganisms in the nineteenth century, and particularly, the work of Lister, Pasteur and Koch, meant that humoral theories of disease came to be challenged. In 1804, there had been 90 patents for medicines in New York but by the middle of the century this number had grown to 1,500. In the US, the 1906 Food and Drug Act was the response to the boom in organic chemistry. From this point forward the ingredients of food and drugs had to appear on the labels and 30 years later a subsequent act went further in requiring that the producer of a medicine specify the use of the medicine. That specification had to be acceptable to the Food and Drug Administration (FDA).

The story of modern antidepressants really began in the early 1950s with the development of the first antipsychotic drug, Chlorpromazine. Roland Kuhn worked on the development of Imipramine under the stipulation that it be considered for use only with endogenous depression.[53] The drug was launched in 1957 but to general ambivalence as a still largely psychodynamic consensus was unable to comprehend how these drugs could help in actually understanding the disease rather than in simply 'curing' the patient. Moreover, depression was a disease that was generally suffered in silence and many were unsure as to whether it would be able to find a market. As such there was generally a paucity of interest in antidepressants at this point.

The emergence of tricyclic antidepressant medication, and the creation by Hamilton of his rating scale for measuring depression, meant that a measure now existed to provide cut-off points in what was then a continuum of normal to abnormal. At this point antidepressant medication (and ECT) was generally considered appropriate for endogenous depression that arose unexpectedly as a result of genetic or constitutional factors. Reactive depression was considered to have resulted from adversity and was still mainly addressed with psychotherapy.

Following the problems with Thalidomide, randomized, placebo-controlled double blind trials became the norm. These trials allowed the testing of the treatment effects of medications that could not be influenced by the expectations of experimenters and would not be influenced by the sample of patients that was chosen for testing. Further, they instituted a comparison of the effects of the medication with groups given placebos in order to try to more accurately discern the effects of the medication. While for some, the use of these trials represented a scientific breakthrough, others derided such a process as it fundamentally ignored important dispositional clinical factors. With regards to the Hamilton scale, many clinicians expressed concern about the use of standardized scores for depression and questioned how relevant such arbitrary, additive symptom scores would actually be to the experience of a patient with depression.[53,55] They were concerned that some symptoms had been given equal relevance to other symptoms that might reasonably have been considered less important to the process of diagnosis. Many felt that, for example, the comparison of early morning waking and feeling suicidal, should not have been given equal importance. Furthermore, the scale (as is the case with subsequent scales like the Beck's Depression Inventory) was very individualistic with many areas of interpersonal functioning neglected. As a result, Hamilton's scale was given little credence for some years until it began to be adopted by the pharmaceutical industry.

The use of randomized controlled trials also worked to reinforce the DSM-III classification criteria and the need to exploit the US pharmaceutical market has provided an impetus for the worldwide adoption of the psychiatric criteria used in the US.

Previously, drugs like antidepressants were considered within the context of what they could reveal about the human psyche, whereas this became less relevant as they were manufactured solely to address mental health relief. That said, the success of Imipramine contributed to the popularity of the catecholamine theories of depression, theories that only began to fade when the Selective Serotonin Reuptake Inhibitors (SSRIs) arrived on the market in the early 1980s.

Antidepressants and the Culture of Cynicism

For a considerable number of years there has been a general lack of public trust associated with biological or physical treatments for depression.[25] There have been a number of reasons for this including a concern over side effects and the quite barbarous history of physical/biological treatments for depression that occurred as recently as the last century. Moreover, many people's concepts of personal responsibility and their belief in the causes and consequences of their condition are also important. As covered in Chapter 2, this particularly western emphasis on personal control and responsibility is pervasive and has led to much of the stigma that currently surrounds depression and some of its treatment options. It is also the case for some that taking an antidepressant can confirm feelings of personal failure and inadequacy as their individual autonomy is transgressed upon.

There are also problems associated with the use, production and marketing of antidepressant medication and to ignore these would be disingenuous. Drug companies have been accused of reinforcing selective interpretations of mental illness and depression in line with financial imperatives and the survival of concepts in the psychological sciences are, to an extent, dependent on the interests with which they coincide. That is not to say that the agenda of the psychological sciences is completely driven by pharmaceutical company interest but their presence and support for a given research agenda undoubtedly contributes to the debates. A drug company can create interest in a given product and sponsor conferences where its use comes under discussion. It can distribute books and journal articles on its efficacy as well as support certain mental health patient groups who are favourably oriented towards the product. The fact that the release of multiple compounds ensures the development of a larger market rather than competing directly with the market share of an initially released product creates a financial imperative that cannot be ignored. To an extent, companies are involved in 'selling' concepts of mental illness and the case of the Monoamine Oxidase Inhibitors is instructive. After work which suggested that they were no greater than placebos for the treatment of depression, they were rebranded, without any clinical evidence, as useful only for atypical depressions. Today this has become an established fact despite there still being insufficient evidence on which to base such a contention.[53]

The editorial boards of many journals are full of individuals who have connections with pharmaceutical companies and many psychopharmacological and biological conceptualizations of depression have come to act like brand names and forms of professional identity through which many professionals in the field unite.

For some people, antidepressant medications like the SSRIs have come to embody the view of human existence as defined by our modern culture of consumption. Happiness is not only a given right but an expectation that has been generated through decades of advertising and consumer products that have aspired to meet all of our needs and desires.[55] There may be some mileage in this idea and there needs to be constant recognition of the more questionable aspects of the pharmacological industry (especially in an era marked by deregulatory fervor). However sometimes, in our rush towards this justifiable cynicism, we forget that antidepressant medication can be enormously effective for people who are experiencing a devastating episode of suffering. It is healthy to be skeptical of such professional interests in the field of depression medication but at no point do I wish to present myself as anti-drugs because I have seen their manifest benefits in too many people who were suffering in agony and desperation.

However, it should be noted that regardless of their efficacy, the structural and socioeconomic factors that can prove so important in precipitating the disease in the first place should not be minimized or somehow marginalized just because we have found an effective treatment at the level of the individual. That we can provide an effective antidepressant medication does not mean that the illness is solely biological nor indeed that it is individual in origin. Such beliefs are popular with a great many people inside and outside of the psychological sciences who have taken the success of antidepressants as an indication of a solely physiological etiology for the illness. Such beliefs are allied to the political ramifications of psychotherapy in their emphasis on the individual, self-based nature of distress and treatment.

I would never tell a person struggling with clinical depression not to take an antidepressant medication but at the same time I would urge that the mental health sciences guard against convenient explanations that follow the logic of 'well if drugs have cured it then the lack of a given compound must be the problem'. Depression is not due to a lack of antidepressant medication in the body. As Horowitz[55] notes, Aspirin helps headaches but headaches are not due to a deficiency of Aspirin. Indeed, the antidepressants are not specific to one disease and have come to be used for depression, anxiety, obsessive compulsive disorder and post-traumatic stress disorder among others. They have come to act as a panacea for a number of different forms of mental suffering and distress and indeed the very term antidepressant has been considered a misnomer in some quarters. It happens that antidepressant medication can be effective at lifting the symptoms for many sufferers but that is not the same as 'curing' depression or the same as addressing what are the root causes of depression in a great many cases.

The individual treatment and social prevention of mental health issues are not incompatible. The problem is that we have failed to strike the right balance and our resources have been disproportionately lent to the former. The many people who suffer from symptoms of depression have little time in modern western culture to fully recover and the pressure to rejoin the workforce has created tighter time constraints for 'recovery'. Hence we have a greater reliance on synthetic agents to hasten the recovery process.

We still do not know enough to categorically and confidently predict the effect that these medications have on the numerous different hormones and neurotransmitters in the brain or how such biological elements relate to genetic and environmental factors. Until we do we should be wary of making grand pronouncements on the meanings attached to medicinal treatments while accepting their virtues for those in often dire need of relief.

Concluding Remarks

Some of the work that I have based my contentions on is the result of the particularly positivistic, individualized approach to behaviour inherent in the modern psychological sciences. As a consequence of my critical stance towards this overly individualistic focus in the psychological sciences, I appreciate the paradox of using such research to substantiate a number of claims and then criticizing the theoretical and philosophical ethos of the discipline. That said, a number of interesting findings have arisen from this work and to reject these findings wholesale would be to discard interesting perspectives on the issue of mental health. It is just important to keep in mind that such an approach has flaws and supports a given political framework for interpreting people and their behaviour.

There is also a paradox at the heart of the treatment that is currently prescribed for clinical depression. There are a great number of professionals who are working tirelessly and often effectively to help to alleviate the profound distress associated with the disease. That said, the political implications of these treatments on a macroscopic scale have contributed to structural conditions that represent depression as an individual illness with an individual genesis. For as long as the mental health industry resides within a framework that speaks the language of self-hood, and minimizes the importance of political and economic forces, it will continue to contribute to the problems that it has been charged with healing.

The political implications of modern day treatments dovetail effectively with the current economic and political structures of the day, especially in the US and the UK. They will continue to receive support and approval as part of a greater structural system that maintains the status quo of resource and power differentials that constrain much of the growing inequality and disempowerment that I have discussed in previous chapters. I am not suggesting a global conspiracy where the movers and shakers in the psychological sciences meet regularly to consider how best they can maintain the power differentials in western society. Rather this system of symbiosis has co-evolved as a number of organizations fail to address the political implications of their actions and perspectives. An insular focus on individuals and individual aspects of distress, on what is treatable, and an unquestioning adherence to the ideological discourses of individualism and consumer-driven self-psychology has led to this effective co-evolution. These are different strands driven by the same cultural and financial imperative not only to help people but to protect the political and financial integrity of the discipline. The political and economic consensus and the mental health sciences collude effectively to create circumstances that suit the protagonists but not always their electorate/patients. Our mental health systems as we know them have grown in conjunction with this Anglo-American capitalism and have come to represent the problem as well as the solution. They are operating to individualize and alienate us. The psychological sciences are under an institutional pressure to stay 'on message' and do so to the detriment of a growing number of people who will become depressed.

The ethos of scientism has combined effectively with the practice of psychotherapy in minimizing the cultural deviation from individualistic capitalist-friendly discourses. Scientific justification and the application of the generic principles of science provide a powerful vehicle with which to mould psychological ideology to the capitalist criteria for success. However, if we are going to apply the discourse of scientism to behaviour and experience then it really is about time that responsibility and accountability were reflected upon. Agendas need to be placed in the open because for as long as they are not visible we will see the perpetual exploitation and misuse of controversial 'scientific' findings.

The process of classifying human behaviours, and the people who exhibit such behaviours, will always be more beneficial for some than for others and such constructions cannot but be the product of ideology. The psychological sciences have privileged access to concepts of mental illness at present and this hegemony requires certain assumptions to be supported, one of which is that individual processes are the source of mental distress. The terms and debates of academic and political discourses operate in order to prevent thought as much as to provoke it. The redundant speculation over the competitive merits of ridiculous dichotomies like the individual versus society or nature versus nurture has been an institutional approach that negates an appreciation that we construct the world in which we live and that we create our truths and rules, values and debates. We are constantly in the process of being negotiated, transformed and represented.

A prominent focus on self-empowerment, self-discovery and self validation will lead to the belief that independence equals empowerment and in reality this could not be further from the truth. Yoga and antidepressants are not effective at the policy level when our individualist psychological constructs replace inadequate childcare, difficult landlords, reduced employment rights and galling poverty.

Chapter 7
Depression and the Future

In the Victorian era, Idiopathic Adrenal Atrophy was the rather grandiose name given to an illness whose principal feature was small adrenal glands. It was only with the passing years that the medical firmament came to realize that this 'condition' actually resulted from the fact that the bodies of the poor were used to teach anatomy.[210] In actual fact, it was the poor who had relatively enlarged adrenal glands in comparison to those who were better off. One might speculate as to why this difference in the size of glands so fundamentally involved in the hypothalamic-pituitary-axis (and, hence with the regulation of stress hormones) persisted, but the difference itself was beyond speculation. Indeed, a new condition was created to account for it.

In much the same way, recent research has led us toward a realization that certain conditions are more likely to predispose some members of society to depression than others and that these differences are also very real. In 1978, Brown and Harris[10] noted that more needed to be done to establish the links between broader economic, political and cultural structures and depression, but there has been very little movement toward accepting this challenge. In 2007, we stand in the same place as Brown and Harris and I echo their sentiments. The last 30 years has taught us that if we do not belatedly recognize this challenge, then a great many more people will succumb to mental distress and depression. Economic circumstances are more difficult now for all but an elite few and it is no longer only those in poverty who are exposed to the vagaries of what we understand to be globalization.

I have considered in detail some of the important political, economic and cultural changes that we have witnessed in the west over the last 30 years. These changes are specific to this period and they have contributed to some enormous difficulties for the people of many countries around the world, not least the countries that witnessed the genesis of the neoliberal project. Our mental health problems are only one symptom of these changes. Anglo-American capitalism and the growing neoliberal consensus is expanding through international corporations, media and political institutions and through the treatment ethos of the psychological and medical sciences.

The centralization of power and commercial imperatives are the major features of the modern institutions that frame our everyday existence and there has been a decline in public service standards, public participation, social capital and democracy. We are an isolated and depoliticized electorate whose options have been constrained by a reduction in the traditional divide between the major political parties. All major political parties now scrap for the crumbs from the centre right political table.

The growing influence of the political and financial elites who sponsor our profit-driven social order is a fundamental component of this globalization. Growing disparities in relative income, greater poverty and poor housing conditions have combined with reduced occupational protection and quality of life to create a growing number of the UK and US population who are experiencing helplessness, reduced social mobility, reduced social networks on which to call on for support and little hope for a future free of these challenges. Freedom has come to be identified as freedom from political and industrial regulations, constraints that would actually benefit a great number of working people.

The multiple effects of such changes are not easy to accurately assess. However, research has suggested that they are invidious and ultimately destructive to our mental health; that this will continue to be so should the current incarnation of globalization continue apace. The mental health industry that has grown around the political framework of recent years has contributed to the problem as well as to the solution. An excessively individualistic focus has led to the personalization of political and structural problems. In combination, this political consensus and individually oriented approach of the psychological sciences has contributed to the manifestation of the individual as an isolated unit of employment with little support from an unrepresentative political process. The elements of the social that interfere with industrial productivity have been sacrificed at the altar of wealth accumulation.

Out of the West

This book has focused on the mental health of the people who live in the developed western world and, specifically, the US and the UK. The reasons for the direction of this focus have already been covered in some detail in earlier chapters. However, the problems associated with globalization and mental health are not limited to the developed countries. In fact, most patients with mood disorders are suspected to reside in the developing world, outside of the realm of effective treatment and significant research attention.[124] In Khartoum, Sudan, 40% of the people had at least one psychiatric disorder and 14% of the people assessed in Calcutta, India, were found to broadly fall within a category of mental disorder. Furthermore, in Rio de Janeiro, Brazil, and Santiago, Chile, it was suggested that 35–45% of the people who responded to a research project were likely cases of mental ill health of some form. Perhaps unsurprisingly, poverty, illiteracy and status as a displaced worker were implicated as significant risk factors for this mental ill health.[124,128]

The sheer extent of the shame, degradation and distress of those in poverty in many parts of the world has not always been appreciated by western medicine and there has been an element of dehumanization[169] in our approach to their suffering. The enormous emotional and psychological distress that many people suffer in the developing world tends to be lost as we focus on the more pressing concerns of keeping as many people alive as possible through the ravages of famine, disease and civil war. However, it has been noted that malnourished children often display a range of symptoms that are difficult to distinguish from depression. Such symptoms as being withdrawn, apathetic, irritable and having low responsivity to stimuli in the environment are symptoms of an institutionalized cycle of interrelated mental and physical health problems, and an appreciation of the scale of mental distress in the developing world is long overdue.

What Can We Do Now?

It is not uncommon to encounter media conjectures that dismiss organizational and structural alternatives to the current political, economic and social consensus as idealistic or somehow railing against the evolutionary 'natural order' of things; a Canute-like presence holding back the inevitable tide of economic progress. However, history has told us that the cultural constructions of a given time and place have tended to be ephemeral, even if this is not always obvious to the prominent thinkers of the time. The great minds of Caesar's Rome might have struggled to consider a world without organized slavery, just as we might struggle to consider economic circumstances where nation states are not slavishly bound to the vagaries of the free market.

In the US, toward the end of the nineteenth century there was a deficit in social capital much like there is now with inequality, crime and degradation rife in the busy cities. The gilded age contained cities that were marked by poverty and disease. Massive corporations that worked to stifle industrial competition set wages for unorganized workers and there was a common concern that a sense of morality and community was disappearing. However, out of this veritable industrial wasteland came a progressive movement for change, organized around the need to oppose the growing influence of the free market and social Darwinism that was so prominent. Civic inventiveness and progressive organization grew between 1870 and 1920 at a rate unmatched previously in the US history.[122]

Settlement movements brought a moral and educational framework to the degraded people who barely existed on the margins of society and a number of groups developed into political forces to campaign for such civil issues like child labour, working men's compensation, stronger antitrust regulation and the length of the working day.[122] The idea of the progressive movement was to create social betterment for the manifest urban problems of the time and the civic nature of the movement was reflected in growing union membership. The point is that a community-driven movement had grown to influence American society to an extent that many would have previously considered unthinkable. This movement had a profound influence on government legislation in a number of areas that improved the quality of life of normal working people.

Recent years have seen huge changes that have affected mental health, physical health, education, housing, consumer protection, child nutrition and health. We have seen a systematic exposure to cynical and forced advertisement and government deregulation in almost all areas of the political and financial spectrum: regulations on which we depend for the protection of our human rights. A great many people have become disengaged with the political process and this has been reflected in recent local and national turn-outs at elections in both the US and the UK. Reagan and Thatcher played a significant role in destroying electoral belief in government, the political process and public services. This is especially true of Reagan who was held up as a role model for many young Americans; this avuncular and benevolent figure who embodied good old fashioned US values.

Of course we cannot lay all of the blame for public cynicism with the political process at the door of Reagan and Thatcher. Indeed, there were changes in the nature of mass leisure, particularly with the arrival of technology that allowed new levels of isolated entertainment to dominate the homes of a growing number of people. This has undoubtedly made it easier to disengage from the political and community processes around which our lives were organized. As modern life in the western world becomes more fragmented and isolated, many people have withdrawn from public affairs and community citizenship, leaving a space that lobbyists and wealthy political groups have not needed two invitations to fill.

Today the sheer cost of the political process has meant that most politicians and political parties have to form relationships with wealthy benefactors whose special interests they are beholden to represent. Such a system is not conducive to the creation of new ideas to address the considerable social and economic difficulties that a growing section of the populous are now facing and which contribute profoundly to their mental health. However, and make no mistake, the way that we engage with the political and economic processes that frame our lives exists in a condition of continual flux. Currently, a great many people have disengaged from the political process and from active citizenship. But as history has shown, such circumstances are only as permanent as they are allowed to be and, while effective changes that work to reverse some of the more harmful effects of the globalization project will take time, they are possible.

Political and Community Initiatives

At the risk of sounding trite, these are difficult times for many people and a noticeable improvement in our mental health is going to require difficult choices. Many believe that this cycle of capitalism is like others before. That it will be followed by a period of social democracy (ala the post-war period). Others believe that our development as a consumer-oriented, free market based society is irreversible and that the social consequences of this transition are also irreversible. Maybe both are true to an extent. Perhaps the near future will bring compromises that allow elements of social democracy to constrain the special interest groups that dominate our political and economic processes. However, the political and economic events of recent years do not fill me with confidence. When Joseph Stiglitz, the former head of the World Bank, and advisor to Bill Clinton, says that the globalization process has been severely manipulated by US corporate interests, we can assume that these negative representations of the globalization project are more than liberal scaremongering.

Changes need to be made to improve and protect the mental health of our families, our friends and ourselves and they need to happen at the macroscopic as well as the microscopic level. That means addressing the social and political structures that frame the inequality and misery to which so many people are exposed. Some of the suggestions below may appear simplistic but then I have never thought that we need to bring the rocket scientists in for this. Many of these prescriptions are not new and can be found in most left-leaning books about why the world is not as nice as it used to be. However, this book is about depression. What is different here is an appreciation that we need to make a number of changes if we are to offer more than partly effective solutions to mental health problems like depression.

An effective global mental health strategy means engaging more people in the political process to work toward an appreciation that this process is fundamental to every important aspect of our lives, from the hours we work, to the mortgages we pay, to the mental and physical illnesses we suffer. This may mean making young American and British citizens undertake mandatory public service in environmental projects, drug clinics or public hospitals.[122] Somehow we have to engage young people with public life and reduce the cynical attitudes that permeate discourses on government and public service. To rebuild a sense of community, we need to reverse the trend of the last 20 years that has seen funding for extra-curricular activities (both school-linked and independent) slashed.

We need to cherish government regulation and use this regulation to reign in the multitudes of special interest groups that have so distorted the political landscape and will continue to do so unless challenged. What we need is a concerted effort to address the structures that promulgate the growing inequality, poverty and misery that so many people experience. From the World Bank income distribution data on a group of 16 OECD countries, there was a clear and marked tendency for greater increases in labour productivity in the more egalitarian countries between the years 1979 and 1990. We need greater political representation and engagement to work toward limiting the extent to which countries around the world increasingly reflect the needs and ideology of Anglo-American capitalism. Economic growth is not the answer to our social problems if the benefits of this growth trickle up rather than down. If we are serious about addressing depression and the mental health needs of our citizens then social justice needs to be placed at the forefront of the political focus. International grassroots community organization needs to ensure that national and international policies on education, employment, taxation and industrial regulation are assessed in terms of their international and collective impact on social equity and quality of life. This movement of democratic forces has to work across more than a handful of nations or else the financial pressure to move toward the Anglo-American model will overpower dissenters. This is uncharted territory but no less necessary because of this. To achieve this we need to address very carefully the many legal advantages that corporations have been given over citizens.

It would mean ensuring a respectable minimum wage indexed to the average wage of a given economy and redistributive tax policies that reduce the growing financial inequality between the wealthy and non-wealthy. It also means restoring the manifest cutbacks in publicly funded health and mental health services that have been a feature of recent years. We need to address our progress on the ridiculous wage discrimination between sexes, an occupational and legislative throwback which is an embarrassment in the 21st century. In general, we need to be constantly aware of strengthening legislation to reduce discrimination and promote real inclusion in school, leisure, work and home.

An effective global mental health strategy also means a global mobilization of shareholders who, in conjunction with governments, have to work toward rejecting the immense corporate salaries that characterize today's corporate elite. We need to create greater awareness of the consumer 'work and spend' treadmill that has become such an established way of life for so many. We know that systematic, organization-wide approaches to reducing work related stress are most effective and so we need to work with employers to convince them of the need for truly flexible working arrangements and lobby the government to ensure that the current movement toward a reduction in job security and the increased casualisation of work is halted and halted fast. We have to focus on innovative ways to mobilize a community ethic in the workplace, such as finding ways to benefit firms that are able to show an improvement in their responsibility to the welfare of their employees.[122] In the UK, the Private Finance Initiative represents an enormous drain of public funds into private concerns and to the detriment of our public services. It either needs to be scrapped or altered in such a way that public representation in such initiatives is sufficiently powerful to be able to protect community concerns.

We need to engender a growing awareness of media representations that lead the public to attribute wealth disparities and welfare status as individual or race-related symptoms of avarice or idleness and appreciate the structural framework that maintains wealth disparities. To move some way to addressing this we need more minorities in the newsroom and audits that address the racial imbalance in both images and content (as was instituted at the Seattle Times in 1988).

With regard to the practice of the political elite leaving cabinet posts to take up well-paid posts on company boards, regulations (that dirty word again) need to be implemented that control the obvious conflict of interest that results from such maneuvering. This is especially the case with regard to companies that have recently benefited significantly from government deregulation policies. Urban planning procedures need to be more carefully monitored and regulated so that the presence of kickbacks to local councils for development permission that is profoundly detrimental to communities is a thing of the past. While we are there, urban planners could focus on more integrated areas of public space that are pedestrian friendly.

Some of the above ideas are not focused, not new and pretty hotchpotch in their aims. I can already hear the accusations of naive idealism but, idealistic or not, we need to be aware of one salient and fundamental fact. If the rising prevalence of depression and psychological distress is to be effectively addressed, these changes need to be made. Persuading the policy makers of the need to invest in strategies to prevent depression is a huge challenge and only time will tell if there is the political or community will to make it happen.

Mental Health Service Initiatives

With regard to the mental health industry and the psychological sciences, a number of key changes will further free our tightly constrained understanding of depression as a dispositional characteristic or illness. There have been some steps in recent years to move toward challenging some of the cherished beliefs and institutions that structure mental health research and teaching; a move to appreciate that all systems exist within a political context that allows specific constructions, reifications, rituals and rules that frame the possession of power within the discipline. The status quo is not always easy to locate, and by accepting the individualistic and intrapsychic paradigm as the way to understand human experience it can sometimes seem like the only way to understand it. However, challenging perspectives exist on the periphery of the discipline and there is a need to move them to the centre of our teaching and research practices in order to enhance our understanding of mental illnesses, the factors that play a role in their etiology and the stigma that so many people experience.

Many of the factors associated with depression are not individual but social and good standards of housing, healthy employment practices and the reduction of inequalities are as important as anything else in the mental health story. The psychological sciences have to face up to their role in this new social capitalism. We need a situationally grounded understanding of how class, sex and race-based power is manifested in the policies and institutions that shape our knowledge and practices.[86] The use of participatory action research, where mental health service users are fundamental to the way that knowledge is constructed and used, is a particularly useful way to address some of the problems in our discipline.

The case management of depression tends to be based around an identification of the patient's needs, the development of a treatment plan and the monitoring of the outcomes of the given treatment plan, and this can prove very effective for some patients whether the treatment used is pharmaceutical or psychotherapeutic. We can still appreciate this utility whist embracing a macroscopic perspective that isolates both structural and individual elements of depression. As mental health professionals we need to be aware of the paradoxical nature of individually-based treatment perspectives and set our research, treatment and policy agendas in relation to the needs of our patients rather than the goals of others who have little interest in mental health issues.

We need to think very carefully about the language used to create our understanding of depression. A dimensional approach rather than a categorical approach could be of great use but we need to retain the vernacular division between feeling a bit down in the dumps and the syndrome that we currently understand as major or clinical depression. If we fail to do this then we will continue to unwittingly perpetuate the profound stigma associated with the illness.

In general, we need to continue to investigate new initiatives to address the stigma of depression because, as things stand, it can still be incredibly difficult to tell friends, family, colleagues or health professionals that we are suffering from depression. To understand the nature of this stigma we need to better appreciate the fundamental notion of personal responsibility that underpins western concepts of being human, particularly in the US. To address this would be going some way to addressing the consultation and treatment problems associated with the illness as well as the enormous sense of alienation that is so much a part of the depressive experience. If a personal crisis can be defined as a set of conditions that present themselves as beyond the coping capacity and resources of the sufferer, then we have to do whatever we can to minimize the institutionally driven nature of the crises that people are exposed to whilst working to increase the resources they have with which to address them. Their resources are profoundly limited if they feel ashamed and weak because they are experiencing mental illness.

I am aware that the numerous suggestions made in this chapter will not eliminate depression from our spectrum of suffering. We will still have depression sufferers and they will still exist in alternating states of unpredictability, perpetual agony and hopelessness. What we might have, however, is fewer of them suffering and for shorter durations. We might not have so many bouts of illness so tied to disenfranchisement and socio-economic disparities, nor have a political process complicit in the genesis and treatment of this suffering.

Depression is a brutal and pervasive illness and a great many of our institutions are complicit in operating without question in a system that makes the illness more and more likely to affect our lives. If we can move toward some of the above changes in politics, business, media and mental health, and increase our appreciation of the importance of the current political and economic structures that frame our lives, then hopefully we can move toward creating new structures. There is such a thing as the public good of countries and societies, and no amount of neoliberal conjecture about personal freedoms and choice can deny this. Consumer inclination has to take a backseat to democratic reason and judgment on matters of human dignity like housing, health and education. When he was president of the board of trade in 1908, Winston Churchill noted a truism, more poignant 100 years on than ever, when he stated that 'the general march toward industrial democracy is not toward inadequate hours of work, but toward sufficient hours of leisure. Working people demand time to look about them, time to see their homes by daylight, to see their children, time to think and read and cultivate their gardens – time in short to live'.[74]

References

1. European Commission Health and Consumer Protection Directorate General. (2004). *Actions against depression.*
2. Chisholm, D, Sanderson, K, Ayuso-Mateos, JL, Saxena, S. (2004). Reducing the global burden of depression. *British Journal of Psychiatry,* 184, 393–403.
3. McNair, BG, Highet, NJ, Hickie, IB, Davenport, TA. (2002). Exploring the perspective of people whose lives have been affected by depression. *The Medical Journal of Australia,* 176(10), 69–76.
4. Greden, JF. (2001). The burden of recurrent depression: Causes, consequences, and future prospects. *Journal of Clinical Psychiatry,* 62(22), 5–9.
5. Wright, A. (1994). Depression. In Pullen, I, Wilkinson, G, Wright, A, Gray, DP (eds.). *Psychiatry and General Practice Today.* American Psychiatric Press.
6. Melfi, CA, Chawla, AJ, Croghan, TW, Hanna, MP, Kennedy, S, Sredl, K. (1998). The effects of adherence to antidepressant treatment guidelines on relapse and recurrence of depression. *Archives of General Psychiatry,* 55, 1128–1132.
7. Schulberg, HC, Magruder, KM, deGruy, F. (1996). Major depression in primary medical care practice: Research trends and future priorities. *General Hospital Psychiatry,* 18, 395–406.
8. Wolpert, L. (1999). *Malignant sadness. The anatomy of depression.* Faber & Faber, London.
9. Parker, G, Manicavasagar, V. (2005). Modelling and managing depressive disorders. Cambridge University Press, Cambridge.
10. Brown, GW, Harris, T. (1978). *Social origins of depression: A study of psychiatric disorder in women.* Routledge, UK.
11. Kuyken, W, Brewin, CR. (1999). The relation of early abuse to cognition and coping in depression. Cognitive Therapy and Research, 23(6), 665–677.
12. Sundquist, K, Gölin, F, Sundquist, J. (2004). Urbanisation and incidence of psychosis and depression: Follow-up study of 4.4 million women and men in Sweden. British Journal of Psychiatry, 184, 293–298.
13. Waraich, P, Goldner, EM, Somer, JM, Hsu, L. (2004). Prevalence and incidence studies of mood disorders: A systematic review of the literature. *Canadian Journal of Psychiatry,* 49, 124–138.
14. Kessler, RC, Berglund, P, Demler, O, Jin, R, Koretz, D, Merikangas, KR, Rush, AJ, Walters, EE, Wang, PS. (2003). The epidemiology of major depressive disorder: Results from the National Comorbidity Survey Replication (NCS-R). *American Medical Association,* 289, 3095–3105.
15. Whybrow, PC. (1997). A mood apart. Picador, London.
16. Parker, G, Gladstone, G, Roussos, J, Wilhelm, K, Mitchell, P, Hadzi-Pavlovic, D, Austin, MP, Hickie, I. (1998). Qualitative and quantitative analyses of a 'lock and key' hypothesis of depression. *Psychological Medicine,* 28, 1263–1273.
17. Kinard, EM. (1982). Child abuse and depression: Cause or consequence. Child Welfare, LXI(7), 403–413.

18. Bifulco, A, Moran, PM, Baines, R, Bunn, BA, Stanford, K. (2002). Exploring psychological abuse in childhood. II. Association with other abuse and adult clinical depression. *Bulletin of the Menninger Clinic*, 66(3), 241–258.

19. Brown, ES, Varghese, FP, McEwan, BS. (2004). Association of depression with medical illness: Does cortisol play a role? *Biological Psychiatry*, 55, 1–9.

20. Penza, KM, Heim, C, Nemeroff, CB. (2003). Neurobiological effects of childhood abuse: Implications for the pathophysiology of depression and anxiety. *Archives of Women's Mental Health*, 6, 15–22.

21. Kristeva, J. (1989). *Black sun: Depression and melancholia.* Columbia University Press, US.

22. Solomon, A. (2002). *The noonday demon.* Vintage, Croydon, UK.

23. Baumeister, RF. (1990). Suicide as escape from the self. *Psychological Review*, 97, 90–113.

24. Jorm, AF. (2000). Mental health literacy. *The British Journal of Psychiatry*, 177(5), 396.

25. Kirsch, I, Moore, TJ, Scorobria, AS, Nicholls, SS. (2002). The Emperor's new drugs: An analysis of antidepressant medication data submitted to the US food and drug administration. *Prevention & Treatment*, 5(23), 1–11.

26. Kadam, UT, Croft, P, McLeod, J, Hutchinson, M. (2001). A qualitative study of patient's views on anxiety and depression. *British Journal of General Practice*, 51, 375–380.

27. Riedel-Heller, SG, Matschinger, H, Angermeyer, MC. (2005). Mental disorders – who and what might help? Help seeking and treatment preferences of the lay public. *Social Psychiatry and Psychiatric Epidemiology*, 40, 167–174.

28. Ellis, PM, Smith, DAR. (2002). Treating depression: The beyond blue guidelines for treating depression in primary care. *The Medical Journal of Australia*, 176(10), s77–s83.

29. Simon, GE. (2002). Evidence review: Efficacy and effectiveness of antidepressant treatment in primary care. *General Hospital Psychiatry*, 24, 213–224.

30. Goldberg, D. (1997). Implications of epidemiological findings for the management of mental disorders encountered in primary care settings. *European Psychiatry*, 12(2), 56–62.

31. Ezquiga, E, Garcia-Lopez, A, de Dios, C, Leiva, A, Bravo, M, Montejo, J. (2004). Clinical and psychosocial factors associated with the outcome of unipolar depresión: A one year prospective study. *Journal of Affective Disorders*, 79, 63–70.

32. Keller, MG, Lavori, PW, Mueller, TI, et al. (1992). Time to recovery, chronicity, and levels of psychopathology in major depression: A 5-year prospective follow-up of 431 subjects. *Archives of General Psychiatry*, 49, 809–816.

33. The ESEMeD/MHEDEA Research Team. (2000). Prevalence of mental disorders in Europe: Results from the European Study of the Epidemiology of Mental Disorders (ESEMeD) project. *Acta Psychiatrics Scandinavia*, 109 (Suppl. 420), 21–27.

34. Pollock, K, Grime, J. (2002). Patient's perceptions of entitlement to time in general practice consultations for depression: Qualitative study. BMJ, 325, 1–6.

35. Pollock, K, & Grime, J. (2003). GP's perspectives on managing time in consultations with patients suffering from depression: A qualitative study. *Family Practice*, 20(3), 262–269.

36. Chew, GCA, May, CR, Cole, H, & Hedley, S. (2000). The burden of depression in primary care: A qualitative investigation of general practitioner's constructs of depressed people in the inner city. *Primary Care Psychiatry*, 6(4), 137–141.

37. Gask, L, Rogers, A, Oliver, D, May, C, Roland, M. (2003). Qualitative study of patient's perceptions of the quality of care for depression in general practice. *The British Journal of General Practice*, 53(489), 278–283.

38. Donoghue, JM, Tylee, A. (1996). The treatment of depression: Prescribing patterns of antidepressants in primary care in the UK. *British Journal of Psychiatry*, 168, 164–168.

39. Cornwall, PL, Scott, J. (2000). Which clinical practice guidelines for depression? An overview for busy practitioners. *British Journal of General Practice*, 50, 908–911.

40. Balestrieri, M, Carta, MG, Leonetti, S, Sebastiani, G, Starace, F, Bellantuono, C. (2004). Recognition of depressión and appropriateness of antidepressant treatment in Italian primary care. *Society of Psychiatry and Psychiatric Epidemiology*, 39, 171–176.

41. Andersson, SJ, Troein, M, Lindberg, G. (2001). Conceptions of depressive disorder and its treatment among 17 Swedish GPs. A qualitative interview study. *Family Practice*, 18(1), 64–70.

42. Dowrick, C, Gask, L, Perry, R, Dixon, C, Usherwood, T. (2000). Do general practitioners' attitudes toward depression predict their clinical behaviour? *Psychological Medicine*, 30, 413–419.

43. Smith, L, Walker, A, Gilhooly, K. (2004). Clinical guidelines on depression: A qualitative study of GPs preferences. *The Journal of Family Practice*, 53(7), 556–561.

44. Andersson, SJ, Lindberg, G, Troein, M. (2002). What shapes GPs work with depressed patients? A qualitative interview study. *Family Practice*, 19(6), 623–631.

45. Grime, J, Pollock, K. (2003). Patient's ambivalence about taking antidepressants: A qualitative study. *The Pharmaceutical Journal*, 271, 516–519.

46. Scott, J, Pope, M. (2002). Non-adherence with mood stabilizers: Prevalence and predictors. *Journal of Clinical Psychiatry*, 63(5), 384–390.

47. Griffith, S. (1990). A review of the factors associate with patient compliance and the taking of prescribed medicines. *British Journal of General Practice*, 40, 114–116.

48. Bucci, KK, Possidente, CJ, Talbot, KA. (2003). Strategies to improve medication adherence in patients with depression. *American Journal of Health-System Pharmacy*, 60, 2601–2605.

49. Schulberg, HC, Pilkonis, PA, Houck, P. (1998). The severity of major depression and choice of treatment in primary care practice. *Journal of Consulting and Clinical Psychology*, 66(6), 932–938.

50. Dwight-Johnson, M, Lagomasino, IT, Aisenberg, E, Hay, J. (2004). Using conjoint analysis to assess depression treatment preferences among low-income Latinos. *Psychiatric Services*, 55(8), 934–936.

51. Stimpson, N, Agrawal, N, Lewis, G. (2002). Randomised controlled trials investigating pharmacological and psychological interventions for treatment refractory depression. *British Journal of Psychiatry*, 181, 284–294.

52. Servan-Schreiber, D. (2004). *Healing without Freud or Prozac*. Rodale, UK.

53. Healy, D. (1997). *The antidepressant era*. Harvard University Press, Cambridge.

54. Cushman, P. (1995). *Constructing the self, constructing America*. Da Capo Press, USA.

55. Horowitz, A. (2002). *Creating mental illness*. The University of Chicago Press, Chicago.

56. Wilson, M. (1993). DSM-II and the transformation of American psychiatry: A history. *American Journal of Psychiatry*, 150, 399–410.

57. Bourdieu, P. (1983). The philosophical institution. In Montefiore, A (ed.) *Philosophy in France Today*, pp. 1–8. Cambridge University Press, Cambridge.

58. Becker, D. (2005). *The myth of empowerment. Women and the therapeutic culture in America*. New York University Press, New York.

59. Raingruber, B. (2002). Client and provider perspectives regarding the stigma of non-stigmatizing interventions for depression. *Archives of Psychiatric Nursing*, 5, 201–207.

60. Sirey, JA, Bruce, ML, Alexopoulos, GS, Perlick, DA, Raue, P, Friedman, SJ, Meyers, BS. (2001). Perceived stigma as a predictor of treatment discontinuation in young and older outpatients with depression. *American Journal of Psychiatry*, 158, 479–481.

61. Pyne, J, Kuc, EJ, Schroeder, PJ, Fortney, JC, Edlund, M, Sullivan, G. (2004). Relationship between perceived stigma and depression severity. *The Journal of Nervous and Mental Disease*, 192(4), 278–283.

62. Dinos, S, Stevens, S, Serfaty, M, Weich, S, King, M. (2004). Stigma: The feelings and experiences of 46 people with mental illness. *The British Journal of Psychiatry*, 184, 176–181.

63. Wedding, D, Niemiec, RM. (2003). The clinical use of films in psychotherapy. *Journal of Clinical Psychology*, 59(2), 207–215.

64. Churchill, R, Khaira, M, Gretton, V, Chilvers, C, Dewey, M, Duggan, C, Lee, A. (2000). Treating depression in general practice: Factors affecting patients' treatment preferences. *British Journal of General Practice*, 50, 905–906.

65. Weich, S, Lewis, G. (1998). Material standard of living, social class, and the prevalence of the common mental disorders in Great Britain. *Journal of Epidemiology and Community Health*, 52, 8–14.

66. Angermeyer, MC, Matschinger, H, Riedel-Heller, SG. (2001). What to do about mental disorder-help-seeking recommendations of the lay public? *Acta Psychiatrica Scandinavica*, 103, 220–225.

67. Goldstein, B, Rosselli, F. (2003). Etiological paradigms of depression: The relationship between perceived causes, empowerment, treatment preferences, and stigma. *Journal of Mental Health*, 12(6), 551–563.
68. Angermeyer, MC, Matschinger, H. (2004). Public attitudes to people with depression: Have there been any changes over the last decade. *Journal of Affective Disorders*, 83, 177–182.
69. Lauber, C, Fulcato, L, Nordt, C, Rossler, W. (2003). Lay beliefs about the causes of depression. *Acta Psychiatrica Scandinavica*, 108, 96–99.
70. Britten, N. (1998). Psychiatry, stigma and resistance. *The British Medical Journal*, 317, 963–964.
71. Lin, E, Parikh, SV. (1999). Sociodemographic, clinical, and attitudinal characteristics of the untreated depressed in Ontario. *Journal of Affective Disorders*, 53, 153–162.
72. Massey, A. (2004). *Beat depression and reclaim your life*. Virgin books. USA (New York).
73. Bauman, Z. (1998). *Work, consumerism and the new poor*. Open University Press, Buckingham, UK.
74. Smith, GD, Dorling, D. (2001). *Poverty, inequality and health in Britain*. The Policy Press, UK.
75. Clarke, P. (2004). *Hope and glory*. Penguin Group, Harmondsworth.
76. Walker, M. (1994). *The cold war*. Arrow Books, London.
77. Theoharis, A. (2004). *The FBI & American Democracy*. University Press, Kansas.
78. Marquand, D. (1997). *The new reckoning. Capitalism, states and citizens*. Blackwell, Oxford.
79. Mitchell, PR, Schoeffel, J. (2003). *Understanding power:* The indispensable Chomsky. Vintage, London.
80. Gray, J. (1998). *False dawn: The delusions of global capitalism*. Granta Books, London
81. Johnson, H. (1992). *Sleepwalking through history: America in the Reagan years*. WW Norton, New York.
82. Ehrman, J. (2005). *The Eighties: America in the age of Reagan*. Yale University Press, New Haven and London.
83. Wilkinson, R. (1996). *Unhealthy societies: The afflictions of inequality*. Routledge, London and New York.
84. Boyer, P. (1990). *Reagan as President*. Ivan R. Dee, Chicago.
85. Schor, JB. (1991). *The overworked American*. Basic Books, London.
86. Bullock, HE, Lott, B. (2001). Building a research and advocacy agenda on issues of economic justice. *Analyses of Social Issues and Public Policy*, 1, 147–162.
87. Vidal, G. (2001). *Imperial America: Reflections of the United States of amnesia*. Clairview, New York.
88. Lott, B, Bullock, HE. (2001). Who are the poor? *Journal of Social Issues*, 57(2), 189–206.
89. Belle, D, Doucet, J. (2003). Poverty, inequality and discrimination as sources of depression among US women. *Psychology of Women Quarterly*, 27, 101–113.
90. Hansen, GB. (1988). Layoffs, plant closings, and worker displacement in America: Serious problems that need a national solution. *Journal of Social Issues*, 44(4), 153–171.
91. Gilmour, I. (1992). *Dancing with dogma: Britain under Thatcherism*. Pocket Books, New York, USA.
92. Evans, EC. (2004). *Thatcher and Thatcherism*. Routledge, London.
93. Lowe, R. (2004). The welfare state in Britain since 1945. Palgrave Macmillian, UK.
94. Winstone, R. (1996). *The Benn diaries*. Arrow Books, UK.
95. Kavanagh, D, Seldon, A. (1989). *The Thatcher effect*. Clarendon Press, Oxford.
96. Radnedge, A. (2006). *One million face being ruined by debt*. The London Metro, May 22nd, 2006.
97. Gilens, M. (1999). *Why Americans hate welfare: Race, media and the politics of antipoverty policy*. University of Chicago Press, USA.
98. Williams, H. (2006). Britain's power elites. The rebirth of a ruling class. Constable, London.
99. Rogers, L. (2005). Thousands join the £1m-plus salary club. The Sunday Times, November 20th, 2005.

100. Sunday Times (2006). *British children among Europe's most deprived*. August 6th, 2006.
101. Ward, L. (2005). *Work smarter not longer, says government*. The Guardian, September 6th, 2005.
102. Monbiot, G. (2000). *Captive state*. Pan Books, London.
103. Grimston, J. (2006). *Supermarkets to carve up the high street*. The Sunday Times, February 19th, 2006.
104. Fox, J. (2001). *Chomsky and globalisation*. Icon books, UK.
105. Stiglitz, J. (2002). *Globalization and its discontents*. Penguin, Harmondsworth.
106. Schirato, T, Webb, J. (2003). *Understanding globalization*. Sage, London.
107. The World Health Organization website. (2006). http://www.who.int (accessed on 21/8/6).
108. The Population Reference Bureau website. (2006). http://www.prb.org (accessed on 21/8/6).
109. Luxemburg Income Study (LIS) Key figures, http://lisproject.org/keyfigures.htm (accessed on 1/8/6).
110. Kay, J. (2003). *The truth about markets*. Pengiun, England.
111. Kennedy, P. (1988). *The rise and fall of the great powers*. Economic change and military conflict from 1500 to 2000. Fontana Press, London.
112. http://www.bbc.co.uk. (2006). BBC news. (accessed on 3/4/6).
113. Foucault, M. (1984). *The Foucault reader*. Pantheon, US.
114. Anderson, S, Cavanagh, J, Hansen-Kuhn, K, Heredia, C, Purcell, M. (1995). No laughter in NAFTA: *Mexico and the United States two years after*. http://www.developmentgap.org/trade/No_Laughter_in_NAFTA.html (accessed on 6/6/6).
115. Benson, J. (1994). *The rise of consumer society in Britain 1880–1980*. Longman, UK.
116. Schor, JB. (2004). *Born to buy*. Scribner, New York.
117. Herman, ES, McChesney, R. (1997). *Global media: The new missionaries of corporate capitalism*. Continuum International Publishing Group. New York (USA).
118. Chomsky, N. (2002). *Media control*. Open Media, New York.
119. Iyengar, S. (1990). Framing responsibility for political issues: The case of poverty. *Political Behaviour*, 12(1), 19–40.
120. Cozzarelli, C, Wilkinson, AV, Tagler, MJ. (2001). Attitudes toward the poor and attributions for poverty. *Journal of Social Issues*, 57(2), 207–227.
121. Bullock, HE, Wyche, KF, Williams, WR. (2001). Media images of the poor. *Journal of Social Issues*, 57(2), 229–246.
122. Putnam, RD. (2000). *Bowling alone*. Simon & Schuster, New York.
123. Platt, S, Martin, C, Hunt, S. (1990). The mental health of women with children living in deprived areas of Great Britain: The role of living conditions, poverty and unemployment. In Goldberg, D, Tantam, D (eds.). *The public impact of mental disorder*. Hogrefe & Huber, Toronto.
124. Harpham, T. (1994). Urbanization and mental health in developing countries; a research role for social scientists, public health professionals and social psychiatrists. *Social Science and Medicine*, 39(2), 233–245.
125. O'Connor, A. (2000). Poverty research and policy for the post-welfare era. *Annual Review of Sociology*, 26, 547–62.
126. Bauman, Z. (1998b). *Globalization: The human consequences*. Polity Press, Cambridge.
127. Caughy, MO, O'Campo, PJ, Muntaner, C. (2003). When being alone might be better: Neighbourhood poverty, social capital and child mental health. *Social Science and Medicine*, 57, 227–237.
128. Bhugra, D, Mastrogianni, A. (2004). Globalisation and mental disorders. *British Journal of Psychiatry*, 184, 10–20.
129. Ustun, TB, Ayaso-Mateos, JL, Chatterji, S, Mathers, C, Murray, CJL. (2004). Global burden of depressive disorders in the year 2000. *British Journal of Psychiatry*, 184, 386–392.
130. Murphy, JM, Horton, NJ, Laird, NM, Monson, RR, Sobol, AM, Leighton, AH. (2004). Anxiety and depression: A 40 year perspective on relationships regarding prevalence, distribution and comorbidity. *Acta Psychiatrica Scandinavica*, 109, 355–375.

131. Klerman, GL. (1988). The current age of youthful melancholia. Evidence for increase in depression among adolescents and young adults. *British Journal of Psychiatry*, 152, 4–14.

132. Rorsman, B, Grasbeck, A, Hagnell, O, Lanke, J, Ohman, R, Ojesjo, L, Otterbeck, L. (1990). A prospective study of first-incidence depression. The Lundby study, 1957–72. *The British Journal of Psychiatry*, 156, 336–342.

133. Munoz, RF, Ying, Y, Bernal, G, Perez-Stable, EJ, Sorensen, JL, Hargreaves, WA, Miranda, J, Miller, LS. (1995). Prevention of depression with primary care patients: A randomized controlled trial. *American Journal of Community Psychology*, 23(2), 199–222.

134. Horwath, E, Weissman, MM. (1995). Epidemiology of depression and anxiety disorders. In Ming, TT, Tohen, M (eds.). *Textbook in psychiatric epidemiology*. Wiley-Liss, New York.

135. Brugha, TS, Weich, S, Singleton, N, Lewis, G, Bebbibgtob, PE, Jenkins, R, Meltzer, H. (2004). Primary group size, social support, gender and future mental health status in a prospective study of people living in private households through Great Britain. *Psychological Medicine*, 35, 705–714.

136. Srole, L, Fischer, AK. (1980). The midtown Manhattan longitudinal study vs. 'The mental paradise lost' doctrine. *Archives of General Psychiatry*, 37, 209–221.

137. European Union Research Group. (2003). *The mental health status of the European population (EUROBAROMETER)*.

138. Lépine, JP, Gastpar, J, Medlewicz, J, Tylee, A, on behalf of the DEPRES Steering Committee. (1997). Depression in the community: The first pan-European study DEPRES (Depression Research in European Society). *International Clinical Psychopharmacology*, 12, 19–29.

139. Katz, SJ, Kessler, RC, Lin, E, Wells, KB. (1998). Appropriate medication management of depression in the United States and Ontario, Canada. *Journal of General Internal Medicine*, 13, 77–85.

140. Bijl, RV, de Graaf, R, Hiripi, E, Kessler, RC, Kohn, R, Offord, DR, Ustin, TB, Vicente, B, Vollebergh, WAM, Walters, EE, Wittchen, H-U. (2003). The prevalence of treated and untreated mental disorders in five countries. *Health Affairs*, 22(3), 122–133.

141. Weissman, MM, Bland, RC, Canino, GL, Faravelli, C, Greenwald, S, Hwu, H-G, Joyce, PR, Karam, EG, Lee, C-K, Lellouch, J, Lépine, J-P, Newman, SC, Rubio-Stipec, M, Wells, JE, Wickramaratne, PJ, Wittchen, H-U, Yeh, E-K. (1996). Cross-national epidemiology of major depression and bipolar disorder. *JAMA*, 276, 293–299.

142. Maier, W, Gansicke, M, Gater, R, Rezaki, M, Tiemens, B, Urzúa, R (1999). Gender differences in the prevalence of depression: A survey in primary care. *Journal of Affective Disorders*, 53, 241–252.

143. Ayuso-Mateos, JL, Vazquez-Barquero, JL, Dowrick, C, Lehtinen, V, Dalgard, OS, Casey, P, Wilkinson, C, Lasa, L, Page, H, Dunn, G, Wilkinson, G, the ODIN Group. (2001). Depressive disorders in Europe: Prevalence figures from the ODIN study. *British Journal of Psychiatry*, 179, 308–316.

144. Lewis, G, Bebbington, P, Brugha, T, Farrell, M, Gill, B, Jenkins, R, Meltzer, H. (1998). Socioeconomic status, standard of living and neurotic disorder. *The Lancet*, 352, 605–609.

145. Brown, GW, Moran, PM. (1997). Single mothers, poverty and depression. *Psychological Medicine*, 27, 21–33.

146. Payne, S. (2006). Mental health, poverty and social exclusion. In Pantazis, C, Gordon, D, Levitas, R (eds.). *Poverty and social exclusion in Britain*. The Policy Press, UK.

147. Lynch, JW, Kaplan, GA, Shema, SJ. (1997). Cumulative impact of sustained economic hardship on physical, cognitive, psychological and social functioning. *New England Journal of Medicine*, 337, 1889–1895.

148. Meltzer, H, Gill, B, Petticrew, M, Hinds, K. (1995). *The prevalence of psychiatric morbidity among adults living in private households. OPCC surveys of psychiatric morbidity among adults living in private households* OCPS, London.

149. Thoresen, RJ, Goldsmith, EB. (1987). The relationship between Army families' financial wellbeing and depression, general well-being, and marital satisfaction. *The Journal of Social Psychology*, 127(5), 545–547.

150. Link, B, Dohrenwend, BP. (1980). Formulation of hypotheses about the true prevalence of demoralization in the United States. In Dohrenwend, BP, Dohrenwend, BS, Gould, MS, et al.(eds.). *Mental illness in the United States: epidemiological estimates*, pp. 114–132. Praeger, New York.

151. Roy-Byrne, PR, Ruso, J, Cowley, DS, Katon, WJ. (2003). Panic disorder in public sector primary care: Clinical characteristics and illness severity compared with 'mainstream' primary care panic disorder. *Depression and Anxiety*, 17, 51–57.

152. Lewis, G, Araya, R. (2002). Globalization and Mental Health. In Sartorius, N, Gaebel, W, Lopez-Ibor, JJ, Maj, M. *Psychiatry in Society*. John Wiley, Chichester.

153. Boardman, AP, Hodgson, RE, Lewis, M, Allen, K. (1997). Social indicators and the prediction of psychiatric admission in different diagnostic groups. *The British Journal of Psychiatry*, 171, 457–462.

154. Lorant, V, Deliege, D, Eaton, W, Robert, A, Philippot, P, Ansseau, M. (2003). Socioeconomic inequalities in depression: A meta-analysis. *American Journal of Epidemiology*, 157, 98–112.

155. Price, RH, Choi, JM, Vinokur, AD. (2002). Links in the chain of adversity following job loss: How financial strain and loss of personal control lead to depression, impaired functioning, and poor health. *Journal of Occupational Health Psychology*, 7(4), 302–312.

156. Galea, S, Ahern, J, Rudenstine, S, Wallace, Z, Vlahov, D. (2005). Urban built environment and depression – A multilevel analysis. *Journal of Epidemiology and Community Health*, 59, 822–827.

157. Chen, YY, Subramanian, SV, Acevedo-Garcia, D, Kawachi, I. (2005). Women's status and depressive symptoms: A multilevel analysis. *Social Science & Medicine*, 60, 49–60.

158. Meyers, BS, Sirey, JA, Bruce, M, Hamilton, M, Raue, P, Friedman, SJ, Rickey, C, Kakuma, T, Carroll, MK, Kiossess, D, Alexopoulos, G. (2005). Predictors of early recovery from major depression among persons admitted to community based clinics. *Archives of General Psychiatry*, 59, 729–735.

159. Van Voorhees, BW, Cooper, LA, Rost, KM, Nutting, P, Rubenstein, LV, Meredith, L, Wang, NY, Ford, DE. (2003). Primary care patients with depression are less accepting of treatment than those seen by mental health specialists. *Journal of General Internal Medicine*, 18, 991–1000.

160. Petterson, SM, Albers, AB. (2001). Effects of poverty and maternal depression on early child development. *Child Development*, 72(6), 1794–1813.

161. McLeod, JD, Shanahan, MJ. (1996). Trajectories of mental health. *Journal of Health and Social Behaviour*, 37, 207–220.

162. Spence, SH, Najman, JM, Bor, W, O'Callaghan, MJ, Williams, GM. (2002). Maternal anxiety and depression, poverty and marital relationship factors during early childhood as predictors of anxiety and depressive symptoms in adolescence. *Journal of Child Psychology and Psychiatry*, 43(4), 457–469.

163. Weich, S, Holt, G, Twigg, L, Jones, K, Lewis, G. (2002). Geographical variation in the prevalence of common mental disorders in Britain: A multilevel investigation. *American Journal of Epidemiology*, 157, 730–737.

164. Kessler, RC, McGonagle, KA, Zhao, S, Nelson, CB, Hughes, M, Eshelman, S, Wittchen, H-U, Kendler, KS. (1994). Lifetime and 12 month prevalence of DSMIIIR psychiatric disorders in the United States. Results from the comorbidity study. *Archives of General Psychiatry*, 51, 8–19.

165. Weich, S, Twigg, L, Lewis, G, Jones, K. (2005). Geographical variation in rates of common mental disorders in Britain: Prospective cohort study. *British Journal of Psychiatry*, 187, 29–34.

166. Priest, RG, Vize, C, Roberts, A, Roberts, M, Tylee, A. (1996). Lay people's attitudes to treatment of depression: Results of an opinion poll for Defeat Depression Campaign just before its launch. *BMJ*, 313 (7061), 858–859.

167. Brown, C, Schulberg, HC, Prigerson, HG. (2000). Factors associated with symptomatic improvement and recovery from major depression in primary care patients. *General Hospital Psychiatry*, 22, 242–250.

168. Kendall-Tacket, KA. (2000). Physiological correlates of childhood abuse: Chromic hyperarousal in PTSD, depression and irritable bowel syndrome. *Child Abuse & Neglect*, 24(6), 799–810.
169. Richter, LM. (2003). Poverty, underemployment and infant mental health. *Journal of Paediatrics and Child Health*, 39, 243–248.
170. Sunday Times September 18th (2005). *Race Chief warns of ghetto crisis.*
171. Weich, S, Twigg, L, Holt, G, Lewis, G, Jones, K. (2003). Contextual risk factors for the common mental disorders in Britain: Multilevel investigation of the effects of place. *Journal of Epidemiology and Community Health*, 57, 616–621.
172. McKenzie, K, Whitley, R, Weich, S. (2002). Social capital and mental health. *British Journal of Psychiatry*, 181, 280–283.
173. Stansfeld, SA, Fuhrer, R, Shipley, MJ, Marmot, MG. (1999). Work characteristics predict psychiatric disorder: Prospective results from the Whitehall II study. *Occupational and Environmental Medicine*, 56(5), 302–307.
174. House, JS, Landis, KR, Umberson, D. (1988). Social relationships and health. *Science*, 241(4865), 540–545.
175. Vinokur, AD, Price, RH, Caplan, RD. (1996). Hard times and hurtful partners: How financial strain affects depression and relationship satisfaction of unemployed persons and their spouses. *Journal of Personality and Social Psychology*, 71(1), 166–179.
176. George, LK, Blazer, DG, Hughes, DC, Fowler, N. (1989). Social support and the outcome of major depression. *The British Journal of Psychiatry*, 154, 478–485.
177. Stansfeld, SA, Fuhrer, R, Shipley, MJ. (1998). Types of social support as predictors of psychiatric morbidity in a cohort of British civil servants (Whitehall II study). *Psychological Medicine*, 28, 881–892.
178. Barkow, K, Maier, W, Ustun, TB, Gansicke, M, Wittchen, HU, Heun, R. (2002). Risk factors for new depressive episodes in primary health care: An international prospective 12 month follow-up study. *Psychological Medicine*, 32, 595–608.
179. Nasser, EH, Overholser, JC. (2005). Recovery from depression: The role of support from family, friends, and spiritual beliefs. *Archives of General Psychiatry*, 111, 125–132.
180. Goering, PN, Lancee, WJ, Freeman, SJ. (1992). Marital support and recovery from depression. *British Journal of Psychiatry*, 160, 76–82.
181. Whisman, MA, Bruce, ML. (1999). Marital dissatisfaction and incidence of major depressive episode in a community sample. *Journal of Abnormal Psychology*, 108(4), 674–678.
182. Yeung, A, Chang, D, Gresham, RL, Nierenberg, A, Fava, M. (2004). Illness beliefs of depressed Chinese American patients in primary care. *The Journal of Nervous and Mental Disease*, 192(4), 324–327.
183. Wilton, RD. (2003). Poverty and mental health: A qualitative study of residential care facility tenants. *Community Mental Health Journal*, 39(2), 139–156.
184. Glied, S, Neufeld, A, McCormack, S. (2003). Women with depression: Financial barriers to access. *Professional Psychology, Research and Practice*, 34(1), 20–25.
185. Weich, S, Lewis, G. (1998). Poverty, unemployment, and common mental disorders: Population based cohort study. *BMJ*, 317, 115–119.
186. Montgomery, SM, Cook, DG, Bartley, MJ, Wadsworth, ME. (1999). Unemployment predates symptoms of depression and anxiety resulting in medical consultation in young men. *International Journal of Epidemiology*, 28, 95–100.
187. Wilson, SH, Walker, GM. (1993). Unemployment and health: A review. *Public Health*, 107, 153–162.
188. Frese, M. (1987). Alleviating depression in the unemployed: Adequate financial support, hope and early retirement. *Social Science and Medicine*, 25(2), 213–215.
189. Anehensel, CS, Clark, VA, Frerichs, RR. (1983). Race, ethnicity, and depression: A confirmatory analysis. *Journal of Personality and Social Psychology*, 44(2), 385–398.
190. Steele, RE. (1978). Relationship of race, sex, social class, and social mobility to depression in normal adults. *Journal of Social Psychology*, 104(1), 37–47.
191. Plant, EA, Sachs, NE. (2004). Racial and ethnic differences in depression: The roles of social support and meeting. *Journal of Consulting and Clinical Psychology*, 72(1), 41–52.

192. Dunlop, DD, Lyons, JS, Manheim, LM, Chang, RW. (2003). Racial and ethnic differences in rates of depression among pre-retirement adults. *American Journal of Public Health*, 93(11), 1945–1952.

193. Miranda, J, Cooper, LA. (2004). Disparities in care for depression among primary care patients. *Journal of General Internal Medicine*, 19, 120–126.

194. Cooper-Patrick, L, Powe, N, Jenckes, MW, Gonzales, JJ, Levine, DM, Ford, DE. (1997). Identification of patient attitudes and preferences regarding treatment of depression. *Journal of General Internal Medicine*, 12, 431–438.

195. Van Ryn, M, Burke, J. (2000). The effect of patient race and socioeconomic status on physician's perceptions of patients. *Social Science and Medicine*, 50(6), 813–828.

196. Gallo, JJ, Marino, S, Ford, D, Anthony, JC. (1995). Filters on the pathway to mental care. II. Sociodemographic factors. *Psychological Medicine*, 25, 1149–1160.

197. Sirey, JA, Meyers, BS, Bruce, ML, Alexopoulos, GS, Perlick, DA, Taue, P. (1999). Predictors of antidepressant prescription and early use among depressed outpatients. *American Journal of Psychiatry*, 156, 690–696.

198. Mechanic, D. (1998). Emerging trends in mental health policy and practice. *Health Affairs*, 17(6), 82–98.

199. Szasz, T. (1988). *The Myth of Psychotherapy*. Syracuse University Press, New York, USA.

200. Stainton Rogers, R, Stenner, P, Gleeson, K, Stainton Rogers, W. (1995). *Social psychology: A critical agenda*. Polity Press, Cambridge.

201. Bowers, J. (1990). All hail the great abstraction: Star wars and the politics of cognitive psychology. In Parker, I, Shotter, J (eds.). *Deconstructing social psychology*, pp. 127–140. Routledge, London.

202. Metzl, J, Angel, J. (2004). Assessing the impact of SSRI antidepressants on popular notions of women's depressive illness. *Social Science and Medicine*, 58, 577–584.

203. Kitzinger, C, Perkins, R. (1993). Changing our minds. *Lesbian feminism and psychology*. New York University Press, New York.

204. Parker, I. (1990). The abstraction and representation of social psychology. In Parker, I, Shotter, J, (eds.). *Deconstructing Social Psychology*. Routledge, London.

205. Billig, M. (1987). *Arguing and thinking: Rhetorical approach to social psychology (european monographs in social psychology)*. Cambridge University Press, Cambridge.

206. Elkind, D. (1998). Behavioural disorders: A postmodern perspective. *Behavioural Disorders*, 23(3), 153–159.

207. American Psychological Association. (2007). http://www.apa.org/about/ (accessed on 18/2/7).

208. University of York Social Policy Research Unit. (2007). *Evaluation of the Employment Advisers in GP Surgeries Pilot*. http://www.york.ac.uk/inst/spru/research/summs/doctor.html (accessed on 31/1/7).

209. Bosely, S. (2006). Depression is UK's biggest problem, government told. Guardian Unlimited. (accessed on 11/10/6).

210. Sapolsky, RM. (1991). Poverty's remains. *The Sciences* (NY Acad Sci), 31, 8–10.

Index